W9-BNA-631

THE
FOUR
DAY
WIN

THE
FOUR
DAY
WIN

END YOUR DIET WAR AND
ACHIEVE THINNER PEACE

Martha
Beck, PhD

RODALE

Notice

This book is intended as a reference volume only, not as a medical manual. The information given here is designed to help you make informed decisions about your health. It is not intended as a substitute for any treatment that may have been prescribed by your doctor. If you suspect that you have a medical problem, we urge you to seek competent medical help.

Mention of specific companies, organizations, or authorities in this book does not imply endorsement by the author or publisher, nor does mention of specific companies, organizations, or authorities imply that they endorse this book, its author, or the publisher.

Internet addresses and telephone numbers given in this book were accurate at the time it went to press.

© 2007 Martha Beck

All rights reserved. No part of this publication may be reproduced or transmitted in any form or by any means, electronic or mechanical, including photocopying, recording, or any other information storage and retrieval system, without the written permission of the publisher.

Rodale books may be purchased for business or promotional use or for special sales. For information, please write to:

Special Markets Department, Rodale, Inc., 733 Third Avenue, New York, NY 10017

Printed in the United States of America

Rodale Inc. makes every effort to use acid-free ♾, recycled paper ♲.

CIP data is on file with the publisher

ISBN-13 978-1-59486-607-4
ISBN-10 1-59486-607-4

Distributed to the trade by Holtzbrinck Publishers

2   4   6   8   10   9   7   5   3   1   hardcover

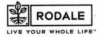

LIVE YOUR WHOLE LIFE™

We inspire and enable people to improve their lives and the world around them
For more of our products visit **rodalestore.com** or call 1-800-848-4735

This book is dedicated to
anyone who has ever felt fat.

CONTENTS

STAGE 3: PREPARATION

ACKNOWLEDGMENTS

The first people I must thank for contributing to this book are my clients, whose stories make my work endlessly interesting, and whose honesty, courage, and openness I admire more than I can say. Y'all know who you are.

I decided to write about this topic through my usual process: bumbling through my own dysfunctions, talking to people I adore, and gradually zeroing in on a topic that made us both swear like pirates and laugh like hyenas. Among these people were: My dear friend Betsy Rapoport, without whose editorial guidance I would be hesitant to write anything at all, and who, as usual, went far beyond the call of duty helping me with this book; my brilliant and hilarious agent, Suzanne Gluck, who took my initial hodgepodge of ideas and unerringly ferreted out the interesting bits; and the fabulous Lisa, who never lets me get away with superficial or half-baked life-coaching claims, and whose energy pushed this project into existence.

Annette Rogers is lavishly gifted with writing talent, compassion, wit, and intellect. She was my first editor on this book, a volunteer subject for various mental and physical exercises. Her editorial feedback is always spot-on, and weirdly, both no-holds-barred and extremely gentle. She's a priceless jewel of a friend, reader, and writer.

Leigh Haber, my editor at Rodale, has been a proponent and advocate for this book since it was just an idea. Her warmth, humor, and laid-back style, combined with her incredible enthusiasm and quickness, made it a pleasure to write this book at about twice the speed my sluggish self would have achieved on its own. Leigh's assistant, Angela Polidoro, has been a gently persistent force guiding *The 4-Day Win* through production.

The fabulous people at *O, The Oprah Magazine,* are my writing coaches, diplomatic constructive critics, and deeply respected colleagues. Mamie Healey is such a gifted writer that having her as an editor is almost too good to be true. Amy Gross's brilliance at spotting an interesting topic, and her generosity in giving me permission to be myself, has helped steer my writing and my life. And every day I thank Gayle King and Oprah Winfrey for creating and running a magazine that challenges me to push the limits of my own thinking.

Lisa Talamini, visionary development director for the Jenny Craig company, jumped into my favorite kind of research before I did. I had a blast working with her to create a product to help dieters psychologically. Norma Hubble and Patti Larchet were equally willing to consider this unorthodox idea, and are simply delightful to know.

My life, not just my career, would be heels-up if not for the stalwart comradeship of Kim Barber, Stacey Shively, and Al Preble. I'm inspired and motivated by their intense curiosity about human change, their insights into the workings of the mind and body, and most of all, their way of taking even the most delicate, distressing psychological dilemma, and turning it into strings of inappropriate jokes.

John Parker, sage and healer, keeps gluing my physical strength back together so that I can actually type words into a computer. He's a source of quiet, peace, strength, and encouragement in a high-pressure life. Also (I sense a theme here) the occasional rude joke.

At the eleventh hour, Bill Baugh jumped into the Web site production for this book with superhuman skill and intelligence. He actually made it *fun*.

Koelle Simpson not only helps run my coaching practice, but has allowed me to benefit from her incredible work with animals. She's wise beyond her years and full of the incongruous insights that pique my curiosity and give me new perspectives on human behavior.

And then, of course, are the people who lighten my life every day. Despite being innocent guinea pigs born into the constant experimentation of my life, my children, Kat, Adam, and Elizabeth, have somehow managed to transform themselves from completely inarticulate 7-pound plasma pets into three of the most amazing people I've ever met. Most of all, I thank my partner Karen, who continues to astound me with her level-headed and compassionate wisdom, and without whom my children and I would all be lost in separate states—not only of the Union, but of despondency, confusion, and neglect.

To all these spectacular individuals, I give my thanks and love. Also unlimited amounts of chocolate. Because that's the kind of diet book this is.

THE
FOUR
DAY
WIN

CHAPTER 1

WHY ARE YOU SO DAMN FAT?

Not that *I* think you are. No, no, no. Why, in those pants, with the light behind you, you look positively willowy. But even if you were large enough to have a gravitational field involving four independent moons, and I happened to notice this (unlikely, since I'm completely blinded by the solar glare of my own self-consciousness), I would never, ever ask you a question as cruel as this chapter title. Nor would you say such a thing to me, were the tables turned. No, you're only that rude and nasty to the one person you can never escape—yourself.

How many times have you accused yourself of excessive heft and inappropriate texture (squishy)? How many times have you asked, "Why am I so damn fat?" I'd try to estimate the number for myself, but I don't think it's possible to count that high. I think that if I programmed my computer to calculate the answer, it would explode.

Anyway, it doesn't matter, because pretty much everyone who asks the question "Why am I so damn fat?" already knows the answer. After all, it's in every magazine and about half the books ever published. While the details of each diet or exercise regimen vary from publication to publication, the basic message of all the vast literature on weight loss is . . . drum roll . . . wait for it . . . this is so exciting . . .

EAT LESS. MOVE MORE.

You're so damn fat because you eat too much and don't exercise enough, right? If you don't already know this, you and I aren't living in the same universe. We've been pelted with weight-loss instruction from the womb.

Some of my friends had parents who offered to pay them for every pound they lost—when they were only *in second grade*. Some were weighed like livestock every morning in front of their families or classmates, but without the merciful follow-up of being immediately slaughtered. Some have circumnavigated the globe, one treadmill session at a time. Some actually paid to have their own jaws wired shut, like volunteer subjects in some barbaric Nazi experiment.

None of these people—not one—is ignorant of the basic principles of weight loss. They're some of the most intelligent, disciplined achievers I've ever met. All of them know many ways to eat less and move more. Is the problem that they lack willpower? Not at all—their willpower is above average. If you've ever stayed on a diet long enough to lose weight, so is yours. No, the problem, for my friends and all the rest of us, isn't that we don't know what to do. The problem is that we don't do what we know. Why not? Contrary to conventional wisdom, the most compelling answer is not in our refrigerators, our restaurants, our mouths, our stomachs, our weak wills, or our basically vile and godless natures. It's in our heads.

THINKING OURSELVES FAT

To get more than a few pounds over our healthiest weight, most of us have to eat more than our bodies really want. True, certain foods make us prone to overeating (dietitians have now proven, in laboratory experiments, that high-fructose corn syrup is the sweat of Satan). But even so, taking in far more calories than we need doesn't physically feel good. After the point when our appetites are sated, we're not increasing physical pleasure; we're overriding physical discomfort. By the same token, environmental factors may invite us to gorge, but they don't actually force us. Your local Burger Binge Bonanza managers may offer all sorts of tallow-laden food, but no one's holding you at gunpoint until you consume every last fry in a king-size super-trough.

Bottom line: Eating is a deliberate behavior, however compelling. Like all deliberate behavior, even if we do it without really thinking about it, the process of eating must be okayed by our brains before it reaches the "action" stage. I know first-hand what it's like to spend years feeling completely out of control in any area connected with food and eating. Many of my clients have been there, too. But we've also seen (and felt) what it's like to be set free from the struggle to control our weight. My experience and research tell me that these liberations didn't occur because we finally found The Right Diet or achieved superhuman willpower. They happened when we learned to operate our minds and thoughts in ways that, science has now proven, literally altered our brains. Why are you so damn fat? At the most fundamental and important level, it's because of the way your brain has been conditioned to operate—because of the way you *think*. And that's what this book is going to help you change.

THERE'S CHANGING YOUR MIND, AND THEN THERE'S *CHANGING* YOUR MIND

I reached the above conclusion after 20 years of intense study, research, and observation on the subject of weight loss. I began as an undergraduate at Harvard, trying to determine why eating disorders, so prevalent in the USA, were almost unheard of in Asia (the answer, I came to believe, isn't physiological, as much as it is philosophical—but we'll get to that later).

The reason this topic appealed to me was that, like many other college students, I had a hell of an eating disorder—and I use the word "hell" advisedly. It started as a simple diet, then morphed into an extended ride on the gain-lose-gain-lose roller coaster. In hindsight, I can see that my attempts to control my body size actually created a syndrome I now call "famine brain," which drew my behavior and attention to eating until my whole life became a struggle with food. This was one of the most horrible things I've ever experienced and is the real reason I'm writing this book. I never want another human being to feel the way I felt when bingeing, dieting, and obsessing about bingeing and dieting constituted my entire psychological universe. It was like one long, hideous visit to the Spanish Inquisition.

As I went on to get my master's and doctorate (also from Harvard, which by some tragic judgment error just kept admitting me), I became fascinated by sociobiology and social psychology, including the psychology of eating. I was particularly interested in the way the mind reacts to eating problems— what, I wondered, was going on in the brains of people like me, people who knew exactly how to stay thin but somehow just couldn't do it? I read everything I could find on the subject. Since no one (at that time) could watch the human brain in action, the answers I found were sparse and incomplete. Still, they were better than nothing, and I began to emerge from weight obsession.

By the time I'd finished my doctorate, I had already become something that probably made my professors roll their eyes and groan: a life coach. Academia was never as exciting for me as was applying social science in the lives of real people; hearing about my clients' lives and watching them change was mesmerizing. In case you're wondering, a life coach is to a therapist as a personal trainer is to a doctor. Psychotherapists work with damaged minds to make them well. I counsel people who are mentally healthy but feel that they could do more with their lives. Since I believe that each person innately knows what his or her "best life" should be, my coaching is all about helping clients tune into their unconscious unrealized dreams, then making those dreams come true.

As I developed more and more effective coaching strategies, I noticed an interesting trend: Many of my clients were dropping excess weight, even though we hadn't talked about weight loss, and they weren't dieting. I began paying more attention to this phenomenon and even wrote a self-help book called *The Joy Diet,* which recommended several small lifestyle changes that I'd found were correlated with weight loss. This led to a joint project with the diet company Jenny Craig, whose wonderful, cutting-edge researchers collaborated with me in creating a DVD that helped their customers with the psychological side of weight loss.

All of these projects were fascinating, but things got even more exciting when computer technology reached a level of sophistication that allowed scientists to create "brain maps," images of the brain at work. Suddenly, scientists could literally map what was happening in the brain of a person with, say, ADD or compulsive cravings. It turns out that certain ways of thinking can literally change the structure of the brain, for example, in ways that make it less prone to craving and more prone to happiness. The implications for weight loss are huge. It's becoming increasingly evident that typical diet strategies actually tell your brain to trigger processes in the body that lead to weight *gain.* Happily, we can reverse that process, repair the damage, and get thin by thinking as well as behaving in specific, often counterintuitive, ways. Would you like to know what those ways are? As luck would have it, that's what this book is all about.

THE 4-DAY WIN PROGRAM

There are two ways you can use the information and strategies you'll find in this book: (1) a thorough course in thought and behavior strategies that will enable you to stay on a healthy-eating program forever with little effort; and (2) a quick fix I call the Jump-Start, which will help you start losing weight immediately. I suggest you use both strategies, though either one alone will help you lose weight. Let's look at the Jump-Start first.

THE JUMP-START: CHANGING YOUR BODY

If you turn to the Appendix of this book, which begins on page 309, you'll find a description of the basic logic behind the 4-Day Win and instructions for following a program that will start changing your body for the better right away. If you follow the program, you'll be thinner in 4 days—perhaps not as thin as you'll end up but noticeably leaner than you were at the outset. That's what adult development theorists call an "early win," and it will help motivate you to continue on the program. *The first 4 days of your weight-loss routine will be the most difficult.* After that, you'll experience an accelerating increase in motivation and success.

THE METAMORPHOSIS: CHANGING YOUR BRAIN

All of this is well and good, but changing your body, exciting though it is, won't be a sustainable transformation unless you also restructure your brain. If you've ever been on a diet or if you're overweight, you almost certainly have neural circuitry in your brain that's programming your body to add and hold on to fat. The astonishing fact that we can change our brains by using our minds and by behaving in new ways (some as simple as breathing differently) is the key to changing this programming. Each chapter of this book contains one or more concrete strategies for transforming yourself into a lean person from the brain outward.

To learn these skills, you could go the very long scenic route that I took: read hundreds of thousands of pages in subjects from nutrition to psychology to physics to animal behavior to philosophy to linguistic epistemology, then spend thousands of hours counseling and observing dieters. But the strategies in this book are designed to take you to Thinland quickly. Some are thought exercises that push your brain to process information in new ways. Others are real-world methods of making healthy living your second nature instead of an unsteady wagon you might fall off at any moment. Each skill is based on a great deal of research, thought, and real-world observation. Did I assemble them in one place because of my love for humanity? Partly. But mostly I did it because of a desire you'll recognize as more powerful and heartfelt: the desire to have thinner thighs.

PUTTING THE JUMP-START
AND THE METAMORPHOSIS TOGETHER

Metamorphosis takes time; caterpillars don't turn into butterflies overnight. It takes weeks to retrain your brain after a lifetime of punishing thoughts about why you're so damn fat. But I know, I know: You have that wedding next week, Uncle Earl's parole hearing right around the corner, and bikini mud wrestling season will be here before you know it—and you want to look good. So I'll give you the best of both worlds. I'll let you leap right into the Jump-Start plan if you promise to come back and stay with me for the rest of the book. Deal?

Deal. We'll work together as if I were coaching you in person. First I'll have you implement the Jump-Start procedure, reading a few chapters to get a little basic understanding of the brain's reaction to dieting, then I'll toss you right into the motivating process of actual weight loss. Once you're losing weight, you'll read the rest of this book, absorbing the explanations and doing the exercises in each chapter. The chapters are short by design. Each one will provide an explanation for some of the problems that inevitably arise in the process of ordinary, willpower-based dieting. Then, I'll take you through an exercise designed to help you internalize the explanation, rewiring your brain and changing your psychological profile so that you'll never need to fall into the wretched, self-reinforcing cycle of typical ineffective dieting ever again.

If you think this means the 4-Day Win will give you more willpower, you're wrong; it will just help you need less. Believe it or not, your willpower is one thing that can't keep you thin. *Basing a weight-loss effort on willpower does the very things to your mind and body that are virtually certain to make you fatter in the long run.* The more time you spend doing traditional dieting, the more trouble you'll probably have keeping weight off, which is what makes it even more vital to undo the physical and psychological damage so that you can be thin and happy. Oh, yeah, did I mention that? If you do this program consistently, you'll end up happy, and not just because you've lost weight.

COLLATERAL BENEFITS

Of course, I know you're not a looks-obsessed dieter; you just want to be a healthy eater. And I'm certain you also watch porn purely for its sophisticated screenwriting. Let's be honest: If you could get chiseled abs by effortlessly trading in a little happiness, you'd do it in a hot second. In a recent study of 4,283 Americans, more than 600 said they'd rather give up *15 years* of their lives than be fat.

According to my life coach philosophy, fat is actually your ally, because if you really want to be lean and if you can only achieve this by becoming fundamentally happier, then the flab you hate will become powerful motivation for overall positive change. Consider it just a felicitous coincidence that each step on the 4-Day Win program will enhance your entire existence, not just improve your body. Losing weight and keeping it off requires that you live an unusually authentic, fulfilling life. I believe it's the mother of all psychological challenges, more difficult than kicking heroin, more delicate than surgery.

As a result, the successful weight-losers I know are incredibly high-functioning people. They've conquered the Everest of issues, and by comparison, most of life's other problems are mere foothills for them. So if you truly want to be lean, and if you can only achieve this by becoming fundamentally happier, your dissatisfaction with your body will be the goad that won't stop bothering you until you create your "right life" or realize your best destiny.

EXERCISE: OPEN YOURSELF TO HOPE

Your exercise for this chapter, like many you'll find in this book, is paradoxically both easy and difficult. I'd simply like you to open yourself to the possibility that, no matter what you weigh, *there is nothing basically wrong with you.*

You may have tried and failed to control your eating many times or continuously over many years. You may have a burdensome past that you believe holds you back from achieving anything, including weight loss. You may have dysfunctional behaviors and traits that you think are making you fat. I believe these failures and dysfunctions are not signs of any inherent defect in your character, but normal reactions to the way our culture views body size and the way most of us try to lose weight. I'm asking you to hope that this is true, to believe that the damage can be undone, and that it is possible to dissolve not only your double chin but many of the problems that have afflicted your self-concept, your relationships, and your ability to achieve any goal.

By the same token, I'm asking you to consider that any discouragement, anxiety, and sorrow you may feel about your body aren't just your tormentors. They're also your teachers, meant to goad you into making your whole life what it's meant to be. The biggest payoff from following the 4-Day Win is the self-evident experience of the fact that none of your pain has been pointless, and no part of your life has been wasted—not one moment. Every mistake you think you've made is part of the foundation on which you can build a life (and a body) that heals, inspires, and delights everyone in your life—especially you. Kidding aside, I truly believe that is why you're so damn fat.

So let's get started.

CHAPTER 2

4 DAYS
AT A TIME

I'm attending Stoneybrook Farms's "Strong Women" convention in Mohonk, New York, where I've met scores of people who've successfully lost large amounts of weight. Some of these fabulous individuals are telling me (because I asked) about the precise events that occurred at the time they stopped putting on fat and started losing it. And I'm hearing the same thing from them that I've heard from other people who have won the weight war.

"Of course, I'd been thinking about it forever," says Lucy, who dropped more than 80 pounds 6 years ago. "I'd been yo-yo dieting since I was a kid. Basically, I'd given up on losing weight, and I was just trying to accept myself and my body. But then I was sick for 4 days, and I noticed my pants were looser. That sort of motivated me. I just started eating less."

"It happened to me on a vacation," says Jane, who has shed more than 100 pounds and wants to lose 20 more. "I went to meet some of my extended family in Eastern Europe. I decided to just enjoy the experience instead of worrying about my weight. My relatives were all big people like me, so I didn't feel like as much of a freak as usual. But I hated the food. When I got back home, after 5 days, my reflection looked thinner than it did when I left. That was the beginning."

"I fell in love with my boss," confesses Sabrina. "We went on a company retreat, and I was so entranced watching him that I kind of forgot about food for once. By the end of the retreat, I could tell I'd lost weight. So I thought, what the heck, I might as well keep going."

"How long was the retreat?" I ask.

"Uh . . . 3—no, it was 4 days, altogether," Sabrina replies.

Four days. Interviewing people about weight loss, I've heard that time frame over and over. Sometimes it's 3, sometimes 5, but the weight-losers I've interviewed keep telling me their turning points occurred in approximately four revolutions of the planet.

It makes sense, when I think about it. For most dieters, it takes about 4 days of calorie restriction to get a slight but noticeable change in body size. That's the early win I described in the last chapter, an observable mark of progress. Adult development experts know that an early win helps enormously for anyone trying to achieve a difficult task by enhancing the sense of self-efficacy that's essential to keep us striving toward distant goals.

EXPLANATION: THE CURIOUS POWER OF THE NUMBER 4

Noticeable weight loss is not the only factor that seems to make a 4-day period significant. I've known for a long time that when I can get a client to do anything consistently for 4 days—writing, exercising, getting up an hour earlier than usual—an internal barrier seems to fall. The new behavior starts to feel normal; life without it seems odd. It takes less discipline to repeat the action.

As I was pondering this one November day, an anchorwoman on CNN reported that the stock market was about to close for Thanksgiving—but only for 3½ days. Wall Street stays up and running until noon every Thanksgiving, she says, because "they don't like to keep the market closed down for 4 days." She doesn't explain why, but I'm convinced it's related to the 4-day weight-loss phenomenon. Four days is the period of time it takes for something to feel like "business as usual." Three-day events are anomalies; something that lasts through that fourth day is a new status quo.

The Rule of 4 seems to be hardwired into the human brain, which comes equipped with a few basic numeric rules. One of these rules is that we can instantly recognize small quantities; if I show you this many dots (. . .) you can see at a glance that there are three of them. But if I show you a few more, say (. . . . . .), you have to stop and count. This is why we break phone numbers into three- or four-digit clumps, a practice called "chunking." Some people can remember chunks of seven units or even more, but the norm is between three and five. Obscure tribes who don't utilize verbal counting still recognize (and have words for) one, two, three, sometimes four, and then many. We have common terms for today, tomorrow, and the day after tomorrow—a 3-day period—but the day after that is just "the future," disconnected from now. Three is a trend, three is the fairy-tale number of king's sons or magic boxes or days before the spell can be broken. Day 4? That's when "happily ever after" begins.

When I started exploiting this little bit of psychological numeracy in my coaching, I found that people who had trouble starting a week-long program of change jumped right in if I asked them to sustain a new behavior for just 4 days. I also discovered that after the 4 days, the inertia that had been keeping them locked into a pattern of action—or inaction—had changed and was now actually pushing them forward. Even though I specified that they were free to stop making a change after the 4-day period, they often said they'd rather continue, because they'd already blasted through the initial resistance and were now starting to see positive change. This happened with so many clients that I began to refer to it as "the 4-day win."

BACK AND FORE: THE TWO KINDS OF SKILLS YOU'RE ABOUT TO LEARN

This book will walk you through many 4-day wins, each of which you can use in two ways: either as a skill to be employed when necessary (like riding a bicycle) or as a habitual behavior you'll do every day (like brushing your teeth). After each chapter, you'll find a model for practicing one specific skill for 4 consecutive days.

The 4-day repetition is necessary to fully install a skill into the hardwiring of your brain. Four daily iterations break through the feeling that you're a novice and make you think of the skill or activity as "something I do." For instance, if you've gone snowboarding, eaten at a certain restaurant, or played poker on just one occasion, and someone asks you about snowboarding or going to that restaurant or playing cards, you'll think, "Yeah, I tried that once." If you've done the activity twice, you still won't think of yourself as "someone who does that," only as "someone who's done that a *couple of* times." After three experiences, you'll probably think and say, "I've done that a *few* times." If you're like most of the people I've quizzed, it's around the fourth iteration that the activity changes in your mind from "something I did a few times" to "something I do." Yes, I snowboard. Yes, I eat at that restaurant. Yes, I play poker.

As you read this book, learning new information and practicing new ways to think and behave, you'll incorporate knowledge into your brain so thoroughly that your way of understanding weight loss, not just the actions necessary to achieve it, will become second nature. Some of the skills you'll learn require daily, habitual action. These are "forefield" skills—they sit in the foreground of your consciousness and your behavior. Other skills you'll learn, incorporate, and then use when they're necessary to get through some barrier or problem; those are "backfield" skills.

Long ago, when I used to cook things, like dinosaurs and pterodactyls, I once made dinner with a group of friends. One woman—I'll call her Roma—came from a wealthy East Indian family and had reached 25 without ever having cooked anything. Ever. The other people in the group had to teach her how to do things we all took for granted, like cracking eggs, pouring ingredients into a bowl, and stirring them with a spoon. Roma was on her way to a degree in higher math from MIT, but your average hamster had more backfield skills in the kitchen.

When it comes to being naturally thin, most modern Americans have similarly lame backfield skills. If you're a chronic dieter, you know the basic eat-less, move-more practices that lead to weight loss, and you try to keep them in the foreground of your mind all the time. But because this way of thinking isn't supported by a host of small but crucial backfield skills meant to help you adjust to various pressures that make you overeat, it never quite "takes." Trying to implement the forefield practices of weight loss without the backfield skills for staying thin is like trying to add eggs to your cake batter without knowing you're supposed to crack them first.

This book will teach you the forefield weight-loss practices you'll need (ways to eat less and move more), but those are almost trivial when compared to learning the backfield skills that will make you a thin person. Each chapter will teach you one technique. Some of these (like being aware of whether you're hungry or full) will come in handy—in fact, are necessary—pretty much every day. Fortunately, they are part of your intrinsic nature, so once you learn them, sustaining them will take very little effort, just a modicum of attention for a little while. The majority of chapters will give you necessary knowledge and teach you a backfield skill, one you won't have to think about until the situation requires it. I'll suggest which backfield skill you'll need for different situations, but once you've learned them, they'll come quite naturally. I suspect you don't think much about how to crack an egg, but when that skill comes in handy, you've got it.

You'll be using a lot of these backfield skills when you create your 4-day wins, especially early in the process of learning to become a thin person. Once you've done a backfield skill for 4 days, you can stop. You may not need to learn every one of these backfield skills. Say you already know how to avoid binge eating. You can skip the "Beating the Binge Monster" 4-day win on page 96. One 4-day win will have established patterns in your brain that will never go away (you can't "unlearn" to ride a bicycle). You'll be able to brush off the rust and pick them up again with confidence whenever you need them.

You'll use your forefield skills in creating a second kind of 4-day win, focusing on things you'll think about and do every day or almost every day. The most important forefield skill you'll employ in a 4-day win is learning to activate a certain way of thinking that I call Thinner Peace. Other forefield skills include modifying your lifestyle so that you'll eat less and move more in ways that will last your whole life, without ever becoming oppressive. I recommend strongly that you do each of these forefield 4-day wins. Most of these skills will come in the last half of this book, and the backfield skills you've already learned will make it much easier to link 4-day wins into a long-term healthy lifestyle.

LINKED 4-DAY WINS

Linking, as opposed to simply learning, is the second way to use your 4-day win skills. You may decide to do a 4-day win that involves, say, doing yoga stretches every day. If you simply learn the moves in 4 days, you'll break through your resistance and become a person who does yoga. If you link five 4-day wins together, you'll have reached a threshold where you'll actually resist *stopping* your yoga practice—it will be easier to sustain it than to drop it. Before you know it, years will have passed, and you'll be a kind of accidental yogi.

I know a group of mountain climbers who scaled a massive cliff face after training on a rock wall that was just over 10 feet high. Their strategy was for one man to climb 10 feet, clinging with his fingernails to ridges no thicker than a credit card. That man would then attach a metal anchor to the cliff, and his companions would use it to haul themselves up to his level. Then a different climber would go up another 10 feet, and so on. The cliff was hundreds of feet high, but none of them ever had to face a solo climb of more than 10 feet.

Breaking a weight-loss effort into 4-day wins is a form of linking climbs, a "chunking" strategy that allows humans to handle any large undertaking. If you have lots of weight to lose, you obviously can't finish the job in 4 days—but if you do all the 4-day wins in this book, you'll have successfully changed your behavior so that your various small victories link easily into a long, natural-feeling, sustained success. Again, you'll not only be able to lose weight; you will literally have changed yourself from a person with weight issues to someone who stays slim naturally and effortlessly. Most weight-loss advice is reversible; if you were a caterpillar, it would just starve you into being a thinner caterpillar. But if you do all the 4-day win exercises, you'll change yourself from a caterpillar into a butterfly. You'll look, feel, think, eat, and behave so differently there will be no fear of going back.

Most of the 4-day wins in this book are simply weapons I want you to have in your weight-loss arsenal. But some are so crucial that to become a thin person, you really need to make them habitual. While these skills are incredibly important, they are often quite simple—for example, mentally repeating a key phrase or leaving a spoonful of food on your plate. Sustaining them, even for the rest of your life, won't require huge investments of time and energy. Gently, sometimes imperceptibly, they'll transform you in ways huge effort never will.

The exercise below will teach you the foundation skill needed to create a 4-day win for yourself. Every other weight-loss skill you master after that will be chunked into 4-day periods.

EXERCISE: CREATING A 4-DAY WIN

STEP 1: PICK A GOAL

Start by identifying any goal you'd like to achieve. Let's start with some weight-related behavior you haven't been able to sustain: exercising every day, not snacking after midnight, consuming at least one daily food item that could imaginably be found in nature. Make sure the goal is *quantifiable*. For example, "Eat more veggies" or "Use butter as a condiment, not a beverage" are too vague to operationalize. "Eat five ½-cup servings of veggies a day" or "Consume no more than 1 tablespoon of butter per meal" are much more useful. Write your goal here:

My Daily Goal: _____

_____

_____

Now notice something that may be so obvious it's invisible to you: This goal isn't useful. How do you know? Because you're not doing it yet. You've been trying to force yourself to do it for some time; if it worked, it would already be a habit. This is all the evidence you need to know that your goal is too big. Next step: Lower your sights.

I operate my entire life, including the writing of this book, by taking what I call "turtle steps." Since I've had lots of disabling health problems over the course of my long, long life, my envisioned goals are usually a lot bigger than my ability to act on them. I'm always trying to level Everest with a hand trowel. A turtle step is a single trowelful of earth, an action that takes me toward my goal but is so easy that I know for sure I can do it. For me, writing a book is an Everest-leveling activity. Writing this paragraph is a turtle step. Now that I've taken it, I must forsooth rest myself awhile. I'll be back tomorrow.

Okay, thanks for waiting. Now I'm taking another turtle step, writing another paragraph. Can working so slowly actually lead to completing anything? You're reading this, aren't you? I'm telling you, tiny steps work. The tortoise usually does beat the hare.

STEP 2: PLAY HALVSIES UNTIL YOUR GOAL IS RIDICULOUSLY EASY TO ATTAIN

So take your first-blush daily goal and cut it in half. (In the case of limiting something rather than increasing it, this means giving yourself permission to decrease your intake, but by only half as much as you think you should. For example, instead of "I will cut 500 calories a day," you'd promise "I will eat 250 fewer calories a day." In reference to the previous examples, you might say, "Eat 2½ servings of veggies a day" or "Consume no more than 2 tablespoons of butter per meal." Then cut *that* goal in half.

Continue lowering your sights until you get to an action step that feels *ridiculously easy,* one you're absolutely sure you can do. If you feel you *should* be able to do something, but the thought of actually doing it leaves you cold or even just a bit chilly, that isn't a turtle step. Picture me sitting across from you, asking you whether you'd be able to commit, heart and soul, to doing this small step. When you get to the point that when I ask you this question ever so earnestly, you'd have to attach lead weights to your eyeballs to keep them from rolling, the step is so damn easy—*of course* you can do this!— then you know you have a turtle step. Write it below.

My Ridiculously Easy Daily Goal: _____

_____

_____

STEP 3: IDENTIFY A REWARD

Now, think of a reward you could give yourself for keeping this goal *today.* I'm not talking about rewards like healthier veins or eventual svelte- ness—you've had those prizes in mind all along, and they've proven insuf- ficient to motivate action. When I say reward, I'm talking about physical objects or pleasurable activities. For instance, today I've decided that I won't snack between breakfast and lunch. My reward for this will be watching a brainless TV show that is presently stored on my Tivo. The very thought of the reward makes me feel slightly perky; I prefer watching that show to munching on a snack I don't really even want.

If you have trouble thinking of a reward, imagine something you'd love to do or own that is either immoral or illegal. Then, modify that reward until it feels slightly wicked but doesn't break any laws or hurt any sentient beings. Since the goal you've set for yourself is modest, you don't have to knock over a bank to reward yourself; allocating 5 bucks to do something somewhat self-indulgent will work. I've had clients choose rewards like dabbing on a favorite perfume or applying a fake 50-cent tattoo just to shock family members. When you think of a reward that feels tempting enough to motivate you to keep the Ridiculously Easy Daily Goal, write the reward here:

My Daily Reward: _____

_____

_____

STEP 4: IDENTIFY A 4-DAY REWARD

Now, think of an additional, slightly larger reward that you'll get if you manage to keep your Ridiculously Easy Daily Goal for 4 consecutive days. *The first 4 days are by far the most difficult part of your new fitness program, so you may have to be quite generous at this stage.* Examples, depending on your bank account, might include buying a cool pair of flip-flops from a discount shoe store; taking time for a matinee movie; getting a babysitter and going out for an actual grown-up dinner with your spouse; having a massage, manicure, pedicure, or any other cure that strikes your fancy. Write your 4-day reward below:

My 4-Day Reward: _____

_____

_____

STEP 5: MAKE SURE THE ACTION AND THE REWARD ARE LINKED

If you meet your ridiculously easy daily goals, you absolutely must give yourself the reward. Same with your 4-day goal. You must also resist any temptation to give yourself the reward if you *don't* meet your goals. If you do all this and you still don't take any action, reduce the task, increase the reward, or do both, until you start moving.

FINALLY . . .

Fill out the form on the next page and post it in at least three places: your bathroom mirror, your refrigerator door, and your car dashboard and/or workspace. Check off each day you manage to complete your ridiculously easy goals.

"My First" 4-Day Win

Ridiculously Easy Daily Goal: _____

Small Daily Reward: _____

_____

Slightly Larger 4-Day Reward: _____

_____

	Dates of My Current 4-Day Win	Check Off Completed Days Here
Day 1:	___ / ___ / ___	_____
Day 2:	___ / ___ / ___	_____
Day 3:	___ / ___ / ___	_____
Day 4:	___ / ___ / ___	_____

If you're like most roundish people, the 4-day win you just designed is focused on the "action" phase of weight loss: eating less and/or moving more. As you read this book, you'll learn why leaping into action like this is actually making you fatter. Oh, you can go ahead and start on the 4-day win you've planned—in fact, the next chapter will lead you to a "jump-start plan" that will mean there's a little less of you, in a good way, 4 days from the moment you start. Just know that I have some very different 4-day wins in mind for you as you start your journey—ones that have nothing to do with eating less and moving more, ones that will help you retrain your brain. You'll end up with a whole new way of thinking, and that is what will ultimately make you into a healthier, more relaxed, and skinnier being.

CHAPTER 3

HOW TO BE SKINNIER IN 4 DAYS

CHANGING YOUR BODY, NOW

Tracy was one of those kids whose mothers and pediatricians put them on the scale, whisper among themselves, and then give happy-face advice about learning to enjoy healthy food, such as raw dandelions, more than unhealthy food, such as food. Before she was old enough to understand the concept of eating less and moving more, Tracy knew that something about her was wrong, unacceptable, excessive.

She tried to fix this. She tried for 50 years. Sometimes she got thinner, and then people were kind to her, and she'd get depressed because it seemed her weight meant more to them than her essential being. Then she'd get fatter and spiral down into real depression because she equated her right to be loved with thinness.

By the time I met her, Tracy's mind and body were both deeply conditioned to repeat this dismal pattern. Tracy herself was about ready to throw in the towel. She joked a lot about suicide, and it didn't really come across as knee-slapping hilarity, if you get my drift.

Tracy and I agreed that she would try a two-pronged approach to changing her body and mind. So we got her a fork with only two prongs—no, we didn't. We approached her new life in two ways: first, with an immediate jump-start plan that began her weight loss immediately; and second, with a program of learning and psychological exercises that changed the whole way she saw her life. That's what this book will do for you.

GETTING THINNER NOW

As I mentioned in the previous chapter, a 4-day win is what psychologists call a forefield skill, something you can plan and do by exerting conscious attention. Using this skill to lose weight requires a little new information, a diet plan, and action. This is all most diet books and counselors have to offer, and it works—in the short run. Without the backfield skills you'll learn here, however, you'll ultimately bounce back up to your old weight (you'll understand this process a lot better once you've read the following chapters).

One way to use this book is to read the whole thing, learning both fore-field and backfield skills, practicing all of them in order, and gradually watching your body get thinner as your mind becomes the mind of a lean person. This may appeal to you if you are the reincarnation of a high Tibetan lama, whose only goal is to reach enlightenment. Otherwise, I recommend using the Jump-Start plan.

EXPLANATION: THE JUMP-START PLAN

If you want to start using 4-day win strategy to lose weight immediately, read Chapters 1 through 10 (hey, don't fuss, you're already halfway through Chapter 3), plus Chapters 20 and 30. Read but don't do the 4-day wins you'll find described there. Turn to the Appendix (page 309) and take the action steps outlined there, which spell out the quickest possible process to get you losing weight. If you follow the instructions in the Jump-Start plan, you'll immediately begin changing your body into that of a skinny person.

However, if you don't read the remainder of the book, understand your Jump-Start plan in its full context, and master the skills presented in each chapter by doing the 4-day wins that most apply to your situation, your brain won't make the same adjustment as your body. It will remain in its current state, and you'll end up like Tracy: a veteran dieter with a brain full of psychological scars and a body full of pretty much anything edible you can find.

To experience a true metamorphosis, not just a one-night stand with your skinny clothes, get to work on the Jump-Start, then read the remainder of this book as the weight comes off. The Jump-Start program will give you a skinny person's body. Reading and internalizing the remainder of the book will give you a skinny person's *life*.

So, if you want to get yourself all Jump-Started, feel free. I'll be right here, waiting for you.

EXERCISE: GIVE YOURSELF A JUMP-START (OR A BREAK)

1. *Read Chapters 1–10, 20, and 30.*
2. *Go to the Appendix and follow the action steps you find there. They will tell you how to get started losing weight now, now, now (though in a patient, Zenlike way).*
3. *Get started on your weight-loss program as instructed.*
4. *Meet me back here in Chapter 3, and go through the chapters in order, doing any 4-day wins as necessary to integrate all the backfield skills you'll need to change your body, brain, and life into that of a naturally and permanently lean human being.*

The interesting thing about Tracy's story is that she was so tired of dieting she decided not to use this Jump-Start plan. Instead, she just learned the skills in this book at a leisurely pace, and guess what? She lost weight without even trying and no longer fears she'll regain it. All the quick fixes and dramatic starvation regimens ever created are pathetically temporary and ineffective next to the transformative power of truly changing your mind, 4 days at a time. So if you're not in hell, and you'd rather lose weight through the gradual process of changing your whole worldview, turn the page and read on. Otherwise, I'll meet you there once your Jump-Start is underway.

"Jump-Start" 4-Day Win

Ridiculously Easy Daily Goal: *I'll read the Jump-Start chapters and follow*

the directions in the Appendix to start losing weight immediately. If I'm not in a

hurry, I'll just read along without Jump-Starting and lose weight in due time as

*I learn my 4-day win practices and skills.*_____

Small Daily Reward: _____

_____

Slightly Larger 4-Day Reward: _____

_____

	Dates of My Current 4-Day Win	**Check Off Completed Days Here**
Day 1:	____ / ____ / ____	_____
Day 2:	____ / ____ / ____	_____
Day 3:	____ / ____ / ____	_____
Day 4:	____ / ____ / ____	_____

If you're already on a weight-loss regimen, remember that the 4-day win will enhance it, not conflict with it. If you know what to do, this program will help you do what you know. Feel free to stay on any weight-loss program while you learn 4-day win skills!

CHAPTER 4

THE TRANS-
THEORETICAL
MODEL
AND THE
PIGGLY WIGGLY
PROBLEM

Every now and again, I'm invited to participate in organized attempts to
help people lose weight—a TV show about dropping those last 15
pounds, a magazine article about keeping New Year's resolutions, that kind
of thing. I'm always brought in to deal with the touchy-feely aspects of weight
loss, while exercise specialists and dietitians handle the hard-core behaviors.
These specialists outline their approaches (eat less, move more) and the dieters listen attentively, as though they've never in all their lives heard any such
thing, though in fact they've been inwardly shrieking these two thoughts to
themselves since the beginning of the Pleistocene Era. Sometimes, I raise my
hand and ask the questions I know the dieters never will.

"I know I *should* eat celery instead of fudge," I'll say, "but what if I really,
really want fudge?"

"Well," say the dietitians and trainers, "you can have a small square of
dark chocolate!"

"But what if I want real fudge? With marshmallows?"

"Oh, you don't keep that kind of thing in the house."

"But what if I sneak out of my house at 3 in the morning and drive to
the Piggly Wiggly and buy a pound of fudge and eat it right at the cash

24

register?" I say. Sadly, this is not a rhetorical question.

At this point, the experts' nostrils begin to flare a little. "Well, you just don't *do* that!" they tell me.

The dieters and I (we will talk about it later) are ashamed. We look at our shoes. We promise ourselves we'll do better. We crave fudge.

This punchy instruction for sticking to a program—"Well, you just *do* it!"—is the psychological strategy offered by almost every diet-and-exercise regimen, especially in the United States. We share a cultural belief that a combination of information and willpower should be enough to ensure compliance with any fitness program. If this worked, America would be a nation of swizzle sticks instead of the pudgiest population in the history of the planet. There's something amiss in our diet strategy. To explain, I shall now turn to a world-class model—not Heidi Klum, but the "transtheoretical model of change."

EXPLANATION: HOW WE CHANGE

In the late 20th century, a couple of researchers named Prochaska and DiClemente analyzed a mass of data from all sorts of social science disciplines, seeking to define the process by which people create transformations in their own lives. They found that successful change proceeds in seven sequential stages: pre-contemplation, contemplation, preparation, action, maintenance, relapse, and termination. These stages make up the transtheoretical model of change, now used in programs to treat addiction, smoking, eating disorders, and other problems all over the world.

The transtheoretical model of change posits that to make lasting change, we have to move through and fully integrate seven stages:

Stage 1: pre-contemplation (I have no intention of changing)
Stage 2: contemplation (I'm thinking of changing)
Stage 3: preparation (I'm getting ready to change)
Stage 4: action (I'm actually making a change)
Stage 5: maintenance (I'm at my goal and holding steady)
Stage 6: relapse (oops, I fell off the wagon)
Stage 7: termination (my work here is done)

The problem with most weight-loss programs is that they try to skip some of the stages, especially the crucial early stages. Skinny experts who design fitness regimens often impose complex lifestyle changes on overweight people the same way the experts themselves might achieve goals in their own lives, such as getting a tattoo or shooting a small, furry, trusting, baby woodland creature. This doesn't require much strategy; you just identify a goal, jump right into Stage 4, take action, follow the rules, finish quickly, then sit back and enjoy the results. Changing from an overweight person into a lean person isn't this simple. It requires permanent, sustained new behavior that alters every aspect of our lives.

Ever since I learned that crocodiles only have to eat about five times a year (did you know that?) I've enjoyed imagining how different human life would be if we, too, went weeks without getting hungry. No lunch dates, no cooking dinner, no midnight trips to the store for bread and milk. Refrigerators and kitchens would probably look very different—you might not even have them in your house. Restaurants would be more like auto-repair shops, where we'd go every few months for a tune-up.

I love to dwell on such things, and not just because I am seriously mentally ill. My social-science training predisposes me to ponder the degree to which human behavior revolves around the issues that helped our ancestors survive natural selection: physical safety, social status, sex, and of course, food. Getting leaner requires transformation at this primordial level, affecting every aspect of our lives. I repeat: this isn't just a quantitative change, like a caterpillar getting bigger. It's a qualitative change, like the caterpillar becoming a butterfly.

Such a transformation requires a full trip through each and every stage of the transtheoretical model. When we go right from pre-contemplation (having no intention of losing weight) to full-bore action (eating less, moving more) we can sustain the effort for a short time—weeks, months, or, in my case, about 20 minutes—but then we slide right back into pre-diet habits. Here's a truth to live by: You can't sustain any significant, voluntary new action without spending adequate time in pre-contemplation, contemplation, and preparation.

You can see this when people are physically forced right into the "action" stage of weight loss. They experience tremendous emotional, logistical, and social upheaval. For example, it's a common misconception that once you've had gastric bypass surgery, losing weight is easy. Anyone who's been through it will tell you this is anything but true. The pounds come off, but the psychological trauma can be apocalyptic—so much so that some patients literally "eat through" the physical limits of their drastically reduced stomachs, suffering horrific pain and medical complications.

The way doctors try to avoid this is to make sure patients spend adequate time thinking about the bypass surgery and its consequences before taking physical action. The irony here is that doing these "thought steps" thoroughly may be enough to sustain change even if you don't have your stomach reduced to the size of a subatomic particle. (Stage 2, contemplation, when done correctly, can literally change your brain until you are a person who never makes midnight trips to Piggly Wiggly—a person who never even *wants* to.) Just as you need to set a broken bone before you can put bandages on the torn skin above it, you must correct the underlying problems before you can fix surface issues (in this case, losing weight).

So this book will teach you how to be thin by covering *all* the stages of change, especially the ones most dieters skip. The vast majority of diet books will propel you directly to Stage 4, giving you detailed instructions about eating less and moving more, right down to the last menu item and squat-thrust. I'm all for that, *as soon as you've mastered Stages 1 through 3*. In later chapters, I'll encourage you to choose a program you like, or create your own program. This book is what you need to successfully implement the program you choose. Again, I'm assuming you know what to do—or can get excellent, detailed advice that will teach you what to do. *This book will enable you to do what you know.*

This book focuses on the psychological and behavioral aspects of change that most diet books never cover: pre-contemplation, contemplation, and preparation. So those stages of change will occupy most of the real estate in the upcoming pages. There'll be a lot less to learn about action, maintenance, relapse, and termination because you can deal with these almost effortlessly once you've internalized all the backfield and forefield skills you'll learn in the first three stages of change.

Even if you're already actively dieting—even if you've had gastric bypass surgery—you'll benefit from the techniques in the upcoming chapters on contemplation and preparation. That said, to lay the groundwork for the chapters to follow, let's see where you are in the transtheoretical model of change right now.

EXERCISE: WHERE ARE YOU?

Determine which of the following statements best describes you:

1. I have no real intention of changing my body or fitness level.
2. I've been thinking about getting more fit, but I haven't actually done

much about it yet. I'm not really sure what I'm going to do, or the best way to go forward.

3. I've decided to lose weight. I've started putting my ducks in a row—reading diet books, signing up at a gym or exercise class, buying healthier food, discussing my plans.

4. I'm currently losing weight. I've changed my eating and exercise habits. It's working, but I still have to focus on it pretty hard. It's a bit (or a lot) of a struggle.

5. I've been doing well on my fitness program for at least 6 months. I've lost some or all of the weight I wanted to lose, and staying fit doesn't require a huge amount of effort. However, I'm still worried about going back to my old habits.

6. I was doing pretty well with my fitness plan, but recently I feel that I'm losing control again. I eat more than I should, exercise less than I should, and I'm worried about regaining the weight I've lost, or gaining even more.

7. I've been doing well on my fitness program for a year or more. I don't even think about it these days. I feel no temptation to eat more than I need to satisfy my real nutritional needs, and I stay active without any particular effort.

Scoring

If you chose number 1, you're in the stage known as
   PRE-CONTEMPLATION.

If you chose number 2, you're in the stage known as
   CONTEMPLATION.

If you chose number 3, you're in the stage known as
   PREPARATION.

If you chose number 4, you're in the stage known as
   ACTION.

If you chose number 5, you're in the stage known as
   MAINTENANCE.

If you chose number 6, you're in the stage known as
   RELAPSE.

If you chose number 7, you're in the stage known as
   TERMINATION.

If you're like most wannabe weight losers, you probably found that you're in Stages 3 through 6. You're definitely not at the first stage, "pre-contemplation," or you wouldn't be reading this, right? Well, maybe. See, the thing is, when you took the quiz on pages 27–28, you probably lied. Not consciously, of course. I'm talking about the invisible force that drives a rather large percentage of your actual behavior: your subconscious mind. Perhaps you're thinking, "Yeah, yeah, I've been pre-contemplating my fat ass since the Reagan administration. I get it. Let's get cracking, Martha." Before you blithely skip the "pre-contemplation" exercises, read the following chapter. To make you feel better, let's call it an exercise and make it your next 4-day win:

"Pre-Contemplative Reading" 4-Day Win

Ridiculously Easy Daily Goal: _Each day for the next 4 days, I'l read through the upcoming chapters on "pre-contemplation."_

Small Daily Reward: _____

_____

Slightly Larger 4-Day Reward: _____

_____

	Dates of My Current 4-Day Win	Check Off Completed Days Here
Day 1:	____ / ____ / ____	_____
Day 2:	____ / ____ / ____	_____
Day 3:	____ / ____ / ____	_____
Day 4:	____ / ____ / ____	_____

If you're already on a weight-loss regimen, remember that the 4-day win will enhance it, not conflict with it. If you know what to do, this program will help you do what you know. Feel free to stay on any weight-loss program while you learn 4-day win skills!

STAGE
1

PRE-CONTEMPLATION

CHAPTER 5

THE POLAR BEAR EFFECT

WHY RESISTANCE IS FUTILE

Try a little experiment for me. For 10 seconds by the clock, think about anything you like, as long as it has no relationship whatever, not even a tangential one, to polar bears. That means no bears of any kind, no furry white rugs, no snow or ice, no igloos, nothing that connects to polar bears in your mind. Got it? Go. 1 . . . 2 . . . 3 . . . 4 . . . 5 . . . 6 . . . 7 . . . 8 . . . 9 . . . 10. Okay, now relax.

So, were you able to keep all polar bear–related thoughts out of your consciousness for the allotted time? Probably not, and even if you managed to keep such thoughts away for 10 seconds, you've had a bunch of them since you stopped trying not to think about them—look, there goes one now. In fact, you've had more thoughts linked to polar bears since you started reading this chapter than you might have had all day—all week, all year—if I hadn't told you not to think them.

This experiment was designed by Daniel Wegner, a Harvard psychologist who studies "the evasion of suppression." Wegner has shown that under any number of circumstances, trying not to think or feel something makes our brains go right to that very thing, whether it's insomnia, performance anxiety, shocking sexual images involving all nine Supreme Court Justices, or a hankering for fried chicken. The harder we try to suppress any mental state, the more our thoughts move into that state, set up camp, open a six-pack, and hunker down for the duration.

This phenomenon is known as the "ironic monitoring process," a label I love because its acronym is "imp." It happens because telling the brain not to think a thought is a paradoxical command. If I ordered you not to keep anything red in your house, and for some unfathomable reason you decided to obey me, the first thing you'd have to do is scurry through your house looking for red things. Your attention would be preferentially drawn to the very thing you were trying to offload. So, when you're dieting strictly, trying very hard not to think about how much you'd love a burrito with spicy marinated chicken and four kinds of cheese melting in golden swirls through an avacado heaven of guacamole with a huge dollop of—sorry. What was I saying?

Oh yes. When you're trying not to think about your favorite gustatory temptations, you'll think about them all the time, in great detail. That's your imp-mind for you.

Wegner's research shows that under ideal conditions, when we're rested, relaxed, and enjoying life, we can suppress thoughts and feelings fairly successfully. But when we have a high "cognitive load," such as stress, annoyance, or time pressure, trying to resist creates "mental states that go beyond 'no change' to become the opposite of what is desired." This means that the more desperately we try to control the plethora of factors that go into losing weight, the more we create a kickback from our brains.

When I ran one of my dieting clients through this exercise, she immediately diagnosed herself with "bi-polar-bear disorder." She'd spent most of her life either suppressing food-related thoughts and behaviors, or experiencing uncontrollable backlash, in which she did nothing but plan menus, shop, cook, and eat. And eat. And eat. This dieting behavior is typical and predictable, given the ironic logic of brain function. And the longer it goes on, the worse it gets.

THE FEEDBACK SCREECH OF DOOM

Since you probably don't give much of a damn about polar bears, the upsurge of bear-related thoughts you experienced at the beginning of this chapter has, in all likelihood, subsided. However, I suspect you care very much about how heavy you are, how you look, and what you eat. The ironic monitoring process means that the more desperate and pressured you feel, the more intrusively you'll brood about (and potentially do) the very things you've sworn off. The higher the emotional stakes, the worse the ironic effects.

Psychologist Stephen Hayes compares this to a "feedback screech" in a microphone. A feedback screech (that earsplitting whine that sometimes happens during a miked performance) occurs when the sound from an amplifier feeds back into the microphone, which sends the sound right back to the amplifier, which makes it much louder and feeds it into the mike again, and so on. Trying to suppress something tends to cause anxiety, which makes the self-suppression more desperate, which makes the ironic effect much worse, which makes us even more upset. . . . If we're worried about not being able to sleep, this can cause epic insomnia. When we're worried about being fat, it can lead straight to consistent overeating or a grand-mal binge. The more you eat, the more you try to stop eating, and the more you try to stop, the more you eat.

I believe America is in the midst of an obesity epidemic not only because we're oversupplied with fattening food, but because *we're telling ourselves we must not eat it.* Check out the cover of any woman's magazine, and what will you see? Articles on dieting, and recipes so fattening that just holding them in your hands causes cellulite to appear on your wrists. Television commercials alternate between ads for weight-loss pills and programs, and ads that promise enormous amounts of food ("Our portions at Munchorama are now too heavy to lift!") This pattern will just continue to escalate, in the individual dieter's mind as in the cultural zeitgeist, because instructions based on resistance and control always trigger psychological and behavioral backlash. In the long run, telling ourselves to go hungry makes us more gluttonous.

PRE-CONTEMPLATION: WHAT WE RESIST, PERSISTS

So if you think you're totally committed to dieting—especially if you're absolutely desperate to get thinner—you are almost certainly your own worst enemy. That impish part of your psyche, the part that keeps you awake when you're worried about getting enough sleep and sends you into brain freeze when you absolutely have to be brilliantly articulate, is already counting the ways in which it plans to scuttle your fitness program. If this makes you hotly indignant or slightly panicky, things are only getting worse. Whatever you are least willing to do, think, or experience is precisely what you're likely to get. It's like one of the baffling equations mathematicians call "strange loops": if you don't try to control yourself, you'll act like a pig, but if you do try to control yourself, you'll act like two pigs, and the harder you try, the sooner you'll end up acting like N pigs, where N is arbitrarily large.

Here's how this relates to the transtheoretical model of change: You may think you've passed the "pre-contemplation" stage, because so much of your psychological energy is focused on resisting your body, your appetite, your habits. But if you're still in a resistance mode, there's a polar bear loose on your neurological property, and it has no intention of letting you starve it. You—the conscious, verbal, thinking part of you—really wants to be thin. But your inner polar bear part wants a burrito, and it's stronger and more persistent than your conscious will. When your "cognitive load" gets a bit too heavy, when you're tired or stressed or sad, the polar bear can easily consume more calories in 5 minutes than you can exercise away in 5 hours.

If any part of you is still in resistance mode, you have to address the issue by going back to "pre-contemplation" and rethinking your approach to weight loss. As part of the 4-day win you found in the previous chapter, take the following quiz. It will help establish how much of your weight-loss efforts are doomed to sabotage by the ironic functions of your impish little subconscious mind.

EXERCISE: CHECK YOUR RESISTANCE TO WEIGHT LOSS

Pre-Contemplation Quiz

Answer the following true/false questions as honestly as possible. Notice that the words "true" and "false" are not always in the same column. Make sure you circle the correct word for each question.

	A	B	
1.	TRUE	FALSE	When I think about my weight-loss program, I feel excited.
2.	FALSE	TRUE	If I can lose weight, I'll get more approval from someone I love.
3.	FALSE	TRUE	I hate the way I look.
4.	TRUE	FALSE	I love the clothes I wear every day.
5.	FALSE	TRUE	I can't stand living in this fat body one more week.

6. TRUE   FALSE   I have lots of loved ones cheering me on in my weight-loss efforts.
7. FALSE   TRUE   I feel nervous or anxious a lot of the time.
8. TRUE   FALSE   I feel comfortable and relaxed eating in front of other people.
9. TRUE   FALSE   No one really notices whether I'm fat or not.
10. FALSE   TRUE   I'm angry at myself for eating so much.
11. FALSE   TRUE   No one's attracted to me when I'm at this weight.
12. FALSE   TRUE   I feel ugly.
13. TRUE   FALSE   I love my body exactly as it is.
14. TRUE   FALSE   I enjoy every bite I eat.
15. FALSE   TRUE   No one really knows how bad I feel about myself.
16. TRUE   FALSE   I believe I'm sexy.
17. TRUE   FALSE   I want to tell everyone about how I'm going to lose weight.
18. TRUE   FALSE   Staying fit is fun for me.
19. TRUE   FALSE   My weight isn't keeping me from being completely happy.
20. FALSE   TRUE   I'm ashamed of myself.

Scoring

Count the number of answers in Column A. Then see where your answers locate you on the following continuum:

0–5 answers in Column A: At a conscious level, you desperately want to lose weight. But subconsciously, you're resisting the process. This doesn't mean there's anything wrong with you, only that you've absorbed negative ideas that will make permanent weight loss virtually impossible for you until you master the "precontemplation" skills you'll find in the next chapters. If you don't learn them somewhere, your weight loss will be difficult and temporary, at best.

6–10 answers in Column A:	You're probably stuck in an oscillating pattern at a weight that's heavier than you want. You manage to lose a few pounds every now and then, but never as much as you'd like. You regain the weight, plus a few extra pounds, whenever you hit a stressful patch in your daily life. The pre-contemplation exercises in this book will help you get beyond this frustrating pattern.
11–15 answers in Column A:	Your weight isn't a horrible issue for you, just an annoying one. You're already doing many of the things that get your subconscious responses past "pre-contemplation," but if you master the exercises at this stage of the 4-day win, you'll be able to stay leaner and feel much better about yourself.
16–20 answers in Column A:	You either started out with relatively few psychological issues around food and weight, or you've done some serious psychological work to become aware of and move past the "pre-contemplation" stage of weight loss. For you, the chapters in this section may already be quite familiar. You might enjoy reading through them as a review, or as validation, but if you feel like moving on to "contemplation" right now, go ahead.

So, how'd you do? If you found you're in high "resistance" mode, you may feel a bit peeved. You may even be experiencing a full-on feedback screech of frustration, perhaps a little feeding frenzy. Don't worry, we can fix that. *But not by going back to your usual dieting methods.* If you're still planning to use those methods, then as Lily Tomlin says, things are going to get a whole lot worse before they get worse. Instead, try this 4-day win:

"Checking for Unconscious Resistance to Weight Loss" 4-Day Win

Ridiculously Easy Daily Goal: _Each day for the next 4 days, I'll test myself_

to see if I'm scoring differently on the "resistance to weight loss" test. If my score is

stable for 4 days, I can be reasonably sure that the results are accurate and work

to overcome any unconscious resistance I may be experiencing.

Small Daily Reward: _____

_____

Slightly Larger 4-Day Reward: _____

_____

	Dates of My Current 4-Day Win	Check Off Completed Days Here
Day 1:	_____ / _____ / _____	_____
Day 2:	_____ / _____ / _____	_____
Day 3:	_____ / _____ / _____	_____
Day 4:	_____ / _____ / _____	_____

If you're already on a weight-loss regimen, remember that the 4-day win will enhance it, not conflict with it. If you know what to do, this program will help you do what you know. Feel free to stay on any weight-loss program while you learn 4-day win skills!

CHAPTER 6

THIS IS YOUR BRAIN ON DIETS

THE FATTENING WAY TO LOSE WEIGHT

Note: If you're on the Jump-Start plan, you've already read this chapter. Glance over it again to see how it fits into the logic of the 4-day win program as a whole. Carry on!

I'm in a gorgeous beach house in Malibu, surrounded by television cameras, crew members, producers, and four delightful women who are the participants in a makeover reality show. The women have been living here for several weeks, being filmed as they go about the business of getting gorgeous. A dietitian prepares fresh meals custom-designed for each woman. A trainer comes to the house to supervise daily workouts. The program is just what most people would think of as an ideal weight-loss setup, and sure enough, it's making the overweight participants thinner, healthier, more physically fit.

And oh, yes, they're also on the verge of a bloody coup. So there's that.

I've come to this show late in the game, since it's my job to help the ladies transition to real life. Right off the bat, I notice that all of them show signs of clinical depression—which is sort of good, because if they weren't so demoralized, I think they would kill their producers. They skulk around the Malibu mansion, staring daggers at the TV personnel, murder in their hollow eyes. Plus, they've been cheating. Last night they were caught ordering pizza from a nearby fast-food restaurant. No one knows what other crimes they may have perpetrated.

"What's *wrong* with them?" a producer asks me. "You'd think they'd be grateful, or at least cooperative. Why would they break rules that are set up for their own good?"

"It's because of the way the brain and body react to food deprivation," I say. "See, when something severely limits our food intake, it triggers a psychological mechanism that . . . "

But the producer's not listening. Like most people, she's absolutely convinced that the recipe for weight loss is intention plus force. She truly believes that to help the makeover gals, she should police them more rigorously, watch them more closely, make it even more difficult for them to get food.

So I give up on the producers and go straight to the dieters themselves. While the cameramen are changing film, we hatch a whispered plot. The next day I send a "care package" by express mail. It's an assortment of board games and jigsaw puzzles, but all the boxes have false bottoms. In the hidden spaces I've packed as many cookies, chocolate, and other forbidden food items as I can. Am I trying to sabotage the women's weight loss? Absolutely not. I'm trying to salvage it. Bet on this: when you see parents basing a kid's allowance on the child's weight loss, or a TV guest announcing her weight-loss intentions to 10,000,000 viewers, you can be pretty darn certain the person in question will end up chubbier. A little evolutionary logic will show you why.

EXPLANATION: FAMINE BRAIN

FACT: Your brain is an astonishingly complex and powerful instrument specifically designed to keep you from losing weight. Your ancestors survived and reproduced because their bodies were incredibly good at conserving fuel as they scurried from cave to cave, seeking edible grubs and possible mates, all, unthinkably, without a single Starbucks within walking distance.

FACT: Because it is an evolutionary imperative, eating is highly rewarding at many levels. Our brains are so attuned to starvation that consuming food causes not only physical satiety, but psychological payoffs. Not eating food makes us hungry, but it also makes us afraid.

FACT: The only natural conditions under which a wild animal will go hungry while exercising strenuously are emergencies—predator attacks, famine, natural disaster, etc.

FACT: Such emergency conditions "turn on" all our psychological and physical responses to stress. This means that dietary restriction and strenuous exercise, especially in combination, cause the brain to fixate on finding food and comfort, while pumping out hormones that signal the body to lay in supplies by becoming more sedentary and storing fat. (Incidentally, this constant bath of stress hormones also leads to a host of awful degenerative diseases.)

FACT: As very socially dependent beings, we get massively stressed out not only by predators and disasters, but also by social conditions such as negative judgment, loss of status, disapproval, and so on. Such factors have been shown to cause sharp rises in stress hormones among various social primates (baboons, chimpanzees, Britney Spears, etc.).

FACT: Sustaining this kind of stress by setting up constraints and expectations that make you even more panicky about keeping your dietary rules triggers your body's famine responses. These responses are far stronger than conscious intention. They are your Survivor instincts: ultimately, they will outwit, outlast, and outplay your attempts to diet by willpower.

FACT: If you increase the pressure to lose weight by swearing before God to go hungry forever, promising on *Oprah* that you'll drop the pounds, or telling your spouse she/he can divorce you if you get above a certain weight, you escalate your stress responses until they make you want to eat everything in the nearest Krispie Kreme distribution outlet, including the cashier. They will also cause your personality to change, much as Linda Blair's character changed in *The Exorcist*.

In short, courting all this stress is *absolutely, positively guaranteed* to cause "Famine brain," the state of mind that is the polar (get it?) opposite of the state of mind you need to lose weight permanently and peacefully. You simply can't outwit Mother Nature.

STARVATION RATIONS

Consider a study published in 1950 by an epidemiologist at the University of Minnesota named Ancel Keys—a study that somehow never gets mentioned in diet books. Keys studied a group of young men who had never worried about their weight and who'd been screened to make sure they were very healthy. Perfect specimens, these guys were; fit, happy, mentally stable.

For 6 months, they restricted their calorie intake by about 50 percent (this is less drastic than many weight-loss programs I've tried, and much less restrictive than the medically supervised fasts some dieters undergo).

After a few months, the men in this study had gone . . . what's the technical term . . . totally barking postal. They were obsessed with food, talking and thinking about it constantly, losing interest in everything else. They were chronically angry, depressed, apathetic, and anxious. They lost their sense of humor. Many began biting their fingernails, smoking, drinking so much coffee that the experimenters had to restrict them to 9 cups a day. They started hoarding, even stealing—not just food, but all sorts of objects. Their relationships suffered. Their hair fell out.

And then there was the bingeing. Several subjects began losing all control and snorking huge amounts of food, then spiraling down into guilt and self-loathing. Some vomited after binges. When the study ended, the binge-ing got worse, not better. For months, many of the men ate between 8,000 and 10,000 calories a day. Many reported feeling *increased* hunger right after a binge. Check out this tidbit from the original study:

> Subject No. 20 stuffs himself until he is bursting at the seams, to the point of being nearly sick and still feels hungry; No. 120 reported that he had to discipline himself to keep from eating so much as to become ill; No. 1 ate until he was uncomfortably full; and subject No. 30 had so little control over the mechanics of "piling it in" that he simply had to stay away from food because he could not find a point of satiation even when he was "full to the gills." . . . "I ate practically all weekend," reported subject No. 26 . . . Subject No. 26 would just as soon have eaten six meals instead of three. (p. 847)

As if this weren't bad enough, the men's metabolic rate (the number of calories it took to sustain their body weight) had dropped an average of 40 percent, illustrating (as a later analyst put it) "the tremendous adaptive capacity of the human body and the intense biological pressure on the organism to maintain a relatively consistent body weight."

This is precisely what was happening to those four ladies in the Malibu reality show, which is why I sent them food. I felt drastic action was needed to stop the escalating starvation response that was already eroding their happiness, causing them to sneak, hoard, and binge. The men in the Keys study gradually returned to something like normal life (although many of them seemed to have permanent behavior problems) *because they stopped trying to restrict their own eating.* Chronic dieters like me, the Malibu Four, and, perhaps, you, may try to restrict our eating for decades on end.

Now that I've corrected the landscape of my brain by using 4-day win strategies, I don't have to restrict my eating, and I no longer suffer from famine-brain's physical and psychological symptoms. Most people assume I've always been thin. But oh, lord, do I remember the hell I imposed on myself by dieting through willpower. Even when I didn't succeed in losing weight, the pressure to eat less made my brain and body fight back like a wild thing. If you've dieted extensively, you, too, have probably wrought havoc on everything from your sex drive to your work performance. Force-based food restriction works for a while, but it always breaks down, and when it does, the starved dieter eats like there's no tomorrow. Try this:

EXERCISE: WATCH YOUR FAMINE BRAIN

As you know, our environment is chock-full of messages that in order to be considered truly beautiful, you must be a small bony object that might easily fit through a subway grate. For just a few minutes, I'd like you to focus your attention on the media messages that really get to you: magazine or TV images of zero-body-fat athletes, dancers, or models; medical reports about obesity and morbidity; the cruel jokes your brothers make about your thick ankles. Write a list of these things in the space below:

1. Messages that make me think I must lose weight: _____

_____

_____

Now, bring to mind the things you tell yourself when you're feeling especially corpulent—perhaps mild exhortations like, "You could stand to trim down," but more likely angry rants, like "You disgusting sack of blubber! No one will ever love you until you lose that hideous flab!" Write these things in the following space:

2. Things I tell myself to make sure I'll lose weight: _____

_____

_____

Now, read over the two lists above. Let these items fill your mind—the skinny models, the angry judgments, the self-hatred. Holding them in your thoughts, answer these questions:

3. With these thoughts in mind, what emotions do I feel?

_____

_____

4. Holding these thoughts in my mind, do I feel more or less desire to eat?

_____

_____

You may have found that you lose all appetite, feeling carefree and delighted during the times you're trying to lose weight through shame and self-admonition. If so, just put this book down and stop eating until you look like Nicole Richie (this will be especially impressive if you are male). If, on the other hand, you are human, you probably just triggered your innate reaction to threats of deprivation. Your brain and body react by giving the order, "Code red, code red! Find fattening food and eat it all and store every bit of it! NOW!"

If you're going to be an effortlessly thin person, this has got to change. In the past, you've probably alternated restrictive regimens with out-of-control eating, more or less like the subjects in the Keys study. This is not because you're a naturally fat person. Absolutely everyone is likely to develop backlash, obsession, and overeating as a physiological response to deprivation. *Overeating and putting on fat is the normal psychological response to the mere expectation of being chronically hungry.* Let me emphasize: not *being* chronically hungry, merely *expecting* to be.

Even if you haven't lost large amounts of weight, this pattern is very likely ingrained into your brain. Just by reading this, you've already begun to change that. The Malibu Four managed to avert disaster—as far as I know, they never killed a producer—but just in case you've reached the level of biological panic I saw when those poor women were at their most desperate, the following chapters will help heal the brain wounds you've innocently inflicted on yourself.

"Observing Famine Brain" 4-Day Win

Ridiculously Easy Daily Goal: *Each day for the next 4 days, I'll watch my own emotional and psychological responses to food limitation, noting where I show signs of famine brain.* _____

Small Daily Reward: _____

_____

Slightly Larger 4-Day Reward: _____

_____

	Dates of My Current 4-Day Win	Check Off Completed Days Here
Day 1:	____ / ____ / ____	_____
Day 2:	____ / ____ / ____	_____
Day 3:	____ / ____ / ____	_____
Day 4:	____ / ____ / ____	_____

If you're already on a weight-loss regimen, remember that the 4-day win will enhance it, not conflict with it. If you know what to do, this program will help you do what you know. Feel free to stay on any weight-loss program while you learn 4-day win skills!

CHAPTER 7

THE BODY
WHISPERER:

GETTING YOUR SUBCONSCIOUS
MIND ON YOUR SIDE

My friend Koelle Simpson, creator of "The Gift of Equus" life-coaching practice, is one of the best "horse whisperers" in the world. Once I saw her work with a horse named Loco, who was so dangerous his owner had been advised to shoot him. Loco reacted to all humans by rearing, kicking, biting, rolling his eyes, and generally acting like a berserk mass murderer . . . until he spent 3 hours with Koelle and turned into a big, sweet, hoofed puppy. Wherever Koelle went, Loco walked quietly right behind her. When she stopped, he'd stand with his nose touching her shoulder, completely content. It would have taken weeks of violent "breaking" by traditional methods to stop Loco's tantrums. I watched Koelle do it in an afternoon, without whips, chains, beatings, rodeo clowns, or any of the other paraphernalia traditionally used to train horses. She didn't even need a rope. Instead, she used movements and body positions that mimicked the way horses instinctively communicate with one another. These movements are so subtle—the angle of the shoulders, a tilt of the head—that many people work with horses and never notice them. But because Koelle has spent years observing and imitating horses, she can now get them to cooperate with her in a way that, while based on evolutionary logic and careful experimentation, seems almost magical.

If you're locked in angry resistance to your own body, if you hate it, if you've ever starved it or forced it to work through exhaustion, you've tried to "break" an aspect of yourself that reacts very much like a wild horse. Your

THE BODY WHISPERER   49

physiology and unconscious instincts may be close to the state Loco was in when I first saw him. If you're deeply committed to this brutal and ineffective strategy, go find a diet book and have at it; I'd like to rat you out to the ASPCA, but they can't prosecute you for torturing your own body. If you're going to use the 4-day win program, however, it's time to learn some body-whispering skills.

EXPLANATION: BODY-BREAKING VERSUS BODY-WHISPERING

We lose weight by gathering information, making rational rules, and imposing them on ourselves with appropriate choices. Mind over matter, right? Of course. It's only logical.

And tell me, how's that working for you?

Probably about as well as traditional horse-breaking techniques worked on Loco—and for all the same reasons. Forcing your rational self's imperatives on your physiology in this way sends a clear message to your body that you don't understand it, don't like it, and fully intend to hurt and deprive it. How could any animal respond to this without panicky resistance? Your instincts fight back by "forgetting" you're on a diet, sneaking Skittles out of the candy bowl on your secretary's desk, ordering secret pizzas like the Malibu Four. At that point, the biggest difference between your behavior and Loco's will be that marginally fewer experts will suggest shooting you, although they may think about it a lot.

The alternative to the ineffective, miserable process of traditional dieting is to befriend your body the way Koelle befriends horses, by communicating with it in a kindly calm way, in a language it understands. We'll discuss this thoroughly in the next few chapters. But for the moment, it will really help if you understand the logic of predator/prey relationships.

THE HUNTERS AND THE HUNTED

Some animals are predators—they kill and eat other animals (a process known as "predation"). Other beasts are purely prey; they don't eat other creatures, but they do get eaten. Predators have built-in attack weapons, like fangs, claws, and eyes located on the front of the head (for stalking). Prey animals have defensive weapons—eyes on the sides of the head (for wider-angle viewing), a herding instinct (there's safety in numbers), and a hair-trigger "flight" response.

Horses, which are prey animals, often feel terrified around us, because they can see we're predators. We approach them with actions that are typical predator behaviors: We fix our eyes on them, we walk straight up to them (horses, because of the position of their eyes, walk in arcs rather than straight lines), we wave our scary, clawlike hands in their faces. Then we tie them up, robbing them of the flight response that is their primary way to feel safe. They go half-crazy with fear, so we add more ropes, maybe a few whips and chains, until they glaze over and give up. We call these horses "broken" for a reason.

Your body, and some aspects of your psyche, react the same way when you use deprivation tactics based on rational control. We humans are both predatory and preyed upon, so we have elements of both animal types in our genetic programming. When it comes to losing weight, the conscious, controlling part of your mind functions like a predator, while the part that resists weight loss has prey-animal responses. Every time you've resisted or forcefully controlled your body's natural inclinations, you've deepened the predator/prey standoff, destroyed a little more of your subconscious's trust in your conscious self. The result: weight war.

This mechanism in human behavior may be what the Chinese philosopher Lao Tzu meant when he wrote, in 2500 BC, "If you want to shrink something, you must first allow it to expand." I don't mean you should let your body go nuts, sucking up premium ice cream until you could break a horse simply by outweighing it. Not at all. I just mean that to lose weight, you must tell your body you're on its side, then give it enough time, space, and kindness to begin trusting you. After that, it will follow you anywhere your mind wants to go. It will keep your rules for healthy eating out of friendship, not fear—and that means it will keep them forever.

INITIATING JOIN-UP WITH YOUR BODY

Koelle's secret is that she speaks fluent Horse—the "language" of body position and gesture that all equine species use to communicate with one another. She began her work with Loco by taking him into a round enclosure, then telling him to run away from her. (The Horse cue for "run," which is understood instinctively by all equines, involves locking eyes, standing with shoulders squared to the animal, and raising your arms with fingers extended. Speaking of irony, this is exactly what most people do to say "Howdy!" when they want a horse to stand still and connect with them.)

Anyway, when Koelle gave the "Run!" cue, Loco immediately started galloping around and around the pen. Koelle walked in a smaller circle, staying behind him, encouraging him to keep running. After a while, Loco started to feel more comfortable—Koelle wasn't lunging at him, and all that running was burning off the adrenaline in his system. Then, since horses need a herd to feel safe, Loco began to consider that this human might be a suitable herd companion. He began giving Koelle signals that he was interested in joining up: locking one ear onto her, licking his lips, bobbing his head. Koelle responded to these polite inquiries by extending Loco an invitation to join up (speaking in Horse, of course, of course). She turned, walked away from him, and stood still with her back to Loco, looking down. What happened next just stuns me every time I see a horse do it: Loco stopped dead in his tracks, then silently walked up and put his head against Koelle's shoulder.

This process is as reliable as it is amazing. All horses do it, even wild ones, if the human can learn to "speak" a bit of Horse with some approximation of accuracy. The first time I stumbled through a join-up and felt the horse's wet-velvet nose touch my shoulder was like nothing I'd ever experienced—with one exception. It reminded me very much of the first time I opened the fridge on my way to a major pig-out, and suddenly realized I didn't feel compelled to eat. After years of dieting, bingeing, overexercising, and wanting to shoot myself, I felt my body decide to join up with me. We've had our arguments since then, but the Loco conflicts never returned. After that, I could choose to eat or not to eat, even when I was very hungry, and my body would come along with the plan.

This entire book is meant to help you "train" your instincts and biology, so that being thin will be a team effort between your mind and its willing ally, rather than its angry, terrified, and seditious prisoner. We'll begin with a few preliminaries that will allow your body to begin regaining its first vestiges of trust in you. This "pre-contemplation" work will get your unconscious mind and your body out of their entrenched resistance patterns.

RUN AWAY! RUN AWAY!

I want to begin this section by telling you what Koelle told Loco: Don't trust me. Don't trust any book, any author, any authority system. If you have dieted before, you almost certainly have "trust issues," because you have starved and attacked the prey-animal side of yourself. So now, trust only your deepest instincts. When you get any piece of advice, including this one, sit with it for a while. See how it makes you feel. *Don't focus on your thoughts—the thinking mind is predatory. Focus on your physical and emotional feelings, without judging or trying to control them in any way.* When you think about a piece of advice, do you feel more trapped or liberated? Do you sense resistance and constraint, as if someone's tied you up, or is there a little more space and freedom to be your true self, feel your true feelings, do what makes you truly happy?

If advice—any advice—makes you feel trapped, don't take it. Not yet. Later, when you feel freer, you may decide it's a grand idea. Until then, stay away from it and do the following exercise instead. *This is the starting point for losing weight at any given moment, no matter how long you've been on a fitness program.* Even if you get skinny as a rail, when life gets stressful, you may go back to overeating. To reverse that trend, do the following exercise. I call it:

EXERCISE: THE 10-MINUTE VACATION FROM PREDATION

Overeating is a self-calming behavior that's triggered by resistance—your resistance to your body's appetites, its resistance to your attempts at controlling it. You can't ask a prey animal to stop being afraid when it feels threatened—everything in its nature makes that impossible. Remember, I'm not just *comparing* your overeating self to a prey animal, I'm telling you it *literally is one.* If you want it to cooperate with you, you must start by helping it feel safe. At least once a day for 4 days follow these instructions:

1. *Find a safe space where you can be uninterrupted for at least 10 minutes. Hints:*
   - Choose a time when you're not hungry. Right after stuffing your face is a good opportunity; your body's animal fear of being hungry will be at its lowest point.

- Find a place where you can be physically comfortable. You can sit or lie down if you like, or it may feel good to move. If so, choose a mindless activity like walking or knitting, rather than something that demands attention, such as cat burglary.
- Make sure you are also *psychologically* comfortable. During the years I was alternately starving and bingeing, I felt safest when I was running or riding a bicycle, which allowed me to obey my "flight" instincts. Nowadays, I get the same comfort from gazing at a wind sculpture outside my bedroom window. It moves, so I don't have to.
- If possible, find a spot where no one can see you, including you (don't sit facing a reflective surface). Being watched makes prey animals very, very uncomfortable.
- Your safe zone should be a place where there's no food visible or readily available. Ideally, it will be a place where nobody eats, ever. At this point in your psychological development, food may confuse or overwhelm your instinctive self.

Keep experimenting until you find a place where your most nervous, paranoid subconscious prey animal can feel as secure as possible. This is the equivalent of taking a horse into the round pen, where it can both run and feel protected by the walls.

2. Stop attacking your body, and start supporting it.

Beating up on yourself when you're already out of control will only leave you emotionally bruised, more crazed, and ultimately fatter. If you want to lose weight, you must drop your predator behavior. That means being supportive, rather than aggressive, toward your body. It won't come naturally at first. You may feel ridiculous. I don't care. Fake it. After you've established a safe place, breathe as deeply and evenly as you can. On each out-breath, tell yourself one or more of the following mantras (you can say them out loud, or do it silently).

- Everything is okay.
- I don't have to do one single thing for the next 10 minutes.
- I can handle this moment, and I don't have to handle anything else.
- My body has suffered a lot. It deserves understanding, not cruelty.

- In the grand scheme of things, how much I eat or weigh matters much less than being kind. I will start by being kind to my body.
- Struggling not to be the person I am right now is pointless and useless.
- If I never changed a thing, the world would keep revolving.
- It's alright to rest.

3. *Wait for signs your body is ready to "join up" with you.*

If you keep silently repeating these thoughts—even if you don't mean them at first—you'll eventually notice a response in your body. It will signal its readiness to accept you as its herdmate with physical cues, like a horse that feels safe enough to join up. Look for these observable signs of the "relaxation response":

- Deep, regular, easy breathing; a sensation of opening in your airway.
- Muscle relaxation, especially in your torso, neck, and shoulders. The space between your shoulders and the crown of your head lengthening.
- Brief spells of laughing or crying (either of these can happen when our fear levels go down; both are ways the body may use to get out of a "fight or flight" state).
- Sleepiness.
- A sense of emotional quiet and peace.
- The taste in your mouth becoming less bitter, more sweet or salty (stress hormones, along with putting fat on you, make your saliva taste bitter).

This skill is its own reward, since it will give you a reprieve from any anxiety or stress you feel in everyday life. It's also the foundation of every other weight-loss strategy, since the fight-or-flight response is what knocks us out of our rational intentions and goads us into overeating, against our better judgment. A 4-day win on this exercise (10 minutes of vacation a day for 4 days) will help you teach yourself to relax, trusting that your body won't freak out as long as you remain focused on calmly experiencing the present moment. Then the instinctive self can stop kicking, rearing, and biting—biting flan, peanut brittle, pork rinds. . . . Repeat this 4-day win until you can create a relaxation response reliably and confidently. Then you'll be ready for the next step.

"Body Whispering" 4-Day Win

Ridiculously Easy Daily Goal: *Each day for the next 4 days, I'll spend 10 minutes in a place where my prey-animal self feels safe. While I'm there, I'll think supportive thoughts, not attacking ones, until I feel a relaxation response.*

Small Daily Reward: _____

_____

Slightly Larger 4-Day Reward: _____

_____

	Dates of My Current 4-Day Win	Check Off Completed Days Here
Day 1:	___/___/___	_____
Day 2:	___/___/___	_____
Day 3:	___/___/___	_____
Day 4:	___/___/___	_____

If you're already on a weight-loss regimen, remember that the 4-day win will enhance it, not conflict with it. If you know what to do, this program will help you do what you know. Feel free to stay on any weight-loss program while you learn 4-day win skills!

CHAPTER 8

THE CREATURE AND THE COMPUTER

Since childhood, Belle's weight has yo-yo'ed repeatedly by as much as 90 pounds. People who knew her at her highest weight often assumed that Belle was weak-willed. Here's how wrong they were: When Belle slipped on a patch of ice and broke her kneecap halfway through her daily fitness hike, she kept walking in agony for 2 miles, basically dragging one leg, rather than violate the rules of her exercise program. On more than one occasion, for several weeks at a time, Belle went on a diet that allowed her to eat nothing but a 400-calorie vitamin soup per day. Somehow, this diet didn't make her feel as peppy as the manufacturer's infomercial had led her to expect. One day, feeling a bit worse than usual, she checked herself into a hospital. The doctor who performed her admittance exam told her she had "the vital signs of a dead woman."

Like most overweight people, Belle had willpower out the wazoo. That's why she had such extreme backlash—remember, however hard you push your brain/body "famine" buttons, that's the force with which they push back. No, Belle did not lack willpower. What she lacked was language skill. Specifically, she had no idea how to communicate with her body, and when her body tried to "talk" to her, she didn't have a clue what it was saying. In general, I've found that the people who struggle the most with weight issues have the poorest mind/body communication. When they learn to speak and interpret their body's language, their physiology finally starts cooperating with their conscious wishes.

56

If you've mastered the basic exercise you learned in Chapter 7, you've learned to call a cease-fire in the war between your mind and body. The exercise in this chapter will help them form a cooperative weight-loss alliance.

EXPLANATION: COMPUTER-CREATURE COMMUNICATION

I've already used a mess of mixed animal metaphors to describe your body, and if you think I'm going to stop now, you are living in a fool's paradise. I'm going to ride that pony for a long, long time, because I'm trying to undo a fatally flawed, infinitely reiterated cultural assumption. Practically all diet experts, and the dieters they advise, have learned to think of the body as a computer, programmed to take instructions from the mind. But only the mind itself acts like a machine. Your body is not a computer. It is a creature.

Not recognizing this obvious fact leads us into huge, frankly stupid, weight-loss mistakes. It makes us struggle uselessly against our instinctive tendencies to eat and store fat, imposing legislated famine until, like its imperative to heal broken bones or repair torn muscle tissue, the body's compulsion to pack on the pounds comes back stronger. Every time.

Your mind speaks computer, and your body speaks creature. The exercise that you completed in the last chapter—taking a "10-minute vacation from predation"—forced your computer-self to memorize and rotely repeat the creature-language words for "I come in peace." That's nice for starters, but if you're ever going to achieve teamwork between mind and body, which you absolutely need if you're going to lose weight, you must learn to understand the messages your creature-self is constantly sending to the computer.

The medium of this communication is not thinking, but *feeling*. This is a mysterious, counterintuitive mode of expression for your computer self. Take Belle, for example. She had the willpower of a Navy SEAL and a genius IQ, but she was unable to do any of these things:

- Notice, understand, and respond compassionately to her own physical pain
- Recognize the sensations of hunger and satiety
- Fully describe her own experiences of fear, anger, grief, or happiness

- Internalize loving feedback from others
- Acknowledge and enjoy her own sexual attractiveness
- Relax both mind and body enough to sleep restfully on a regular basis

It never ceases to amaze me how many brilliant people lack these basic skills, all of which my beagle has in spades (I'm just guessing on the "sexual attractiveness" part, but he can certainly strut like a stud). When I work with severely overweight clients, I often have the impression that they wouldn't notice if I performed a tonsillectomy on them while we chatted. They literally can't tell me whether they're hot or cold, tired or wired, comfortable or uncomfortable. They don't know. I understand this, because I used to be like them. Twice, during my weight-war days, I got frostbite from failing to notice severe cold (once while standing outside in the snow and once while packed in medical ice bags at a physical therapist's office). On another occasion, when I was working with sharp-pointed technical pens, I stood up and walked across a room before noticing that one of the pens was sticking out of my thigh like the hypodermic lodged in Uma Thurman's chest in *Pulp Fiction*.

Such obliviousness to feeling is very useful when we're running from predators, and I strongly encourage you to use it the next time you're attacked by wolves. I encourage you even more strongly to *stop* using it once the wolves are gone, because if you don't, you'll end up with heart disease, high blood pressure, panic attacks, and enough body fat to fuel a midsize oil-burning generator for at least one fiscal quarter. Traditional dieting relies on your ability to go numb to, or at the very least override, your physical and emotional feelings. This will make you feel focused, exhilarated, in command and in control, right up until the moment the polar-bear effect kicks in, and you accidentally eat the snack food aisle at your local Wal-Mart.

The exercise you're about to learn will start you on the road to paying close, appreciative attention to your own feelings. Helpful hint: If you have no idea what you're feeling emotionally, you can always get there by exploring what you're feeling physically. It's impossible to experience an emotion without creating a physical trace in your body. Your computer-mind will ignore, twist, deny, and project interpretations of the world as it blindly run its programmed ideas about weight loss, because the mind (and I say this with all due respect) has the constancy and reliability of a crack whore. Your body, on the other hand—the body you hate, malign, and torture—is, to quote Shakespeare, "as true as truest horse." Listening to it is your only ticket out of Fatsville.

I remember my father sitting at our Thanksgiving dinner, telling our large and boisterous family that we should stay on the alert for the two key signals that we'd eaten enough. First, he said, we would see a blinding flash. Second, everything would go dark. At that point, my father advised, we might want to stop forcing down mashed potatoes and start on the pie.

For those of us with teensy weensy little weight obsessions, this isn't all that much of an exaggeration. Consider the person who ate 19 pounds of food, including about 3 pounds of meat and 10 pounds of healthy fruits and vegetables, before dying of a ruptured stomach. Was this person a strapping, 7-foot-tall lumberjack who'd just leveled the forests of Canada with a hand ax? No. It was a 23-year-old fashion model. As such, she'd probably kept her body weight far too low, and gone far too hungry, for so long that she'd lost all awareness of the sensations that are supposed to regulate food consumption.

Allowed to function as nature intended, your creature-self will stop eating when two conditions are met: 1) it senses that you aren't hungry any more (not that you're full, but that you're simply not hungry); and 2) it's confident there will be no food shortage in the foreseeable future. We'll talk about condition 2 later on in this book, though you may already have noticed that it runs contrary to the whole idea of righteous self-deprivation as a weight-control strategy. Right now, we're concerned with condition 1. To stop eating before you've consumed too much food for your system, you need to know and respond to fairly subtle signals sent by your creature-self to your computerlike brain. Here's how.

EXERCISE: SENSATION INTERPRETATION:

Learning To Speak "Creature"

1. *Start by going on your "10-minute vacation from predation" and establish a good, strong relaxation response. It's best to do this when you've just eaten, because to do the exercise, you need to go without food for the next 15 minutes.*

If you're unable to do this, go back to the exercise in Chapter 5, and do another 4-day win. Then try this exercise again. Going forward without getting to the point where your body starts to relax is like trying to pour water when it's frozen solid. You can only "melt" your rigid dietary habits by relaxing.

2. *Describe, in very precise words, the sensations in your hands and feet.*

We're starting with hands and feet because they're the parts of the body that usually frighten chubby people the least. Even so, you may be so used to ignoring your body's sensations that this simple-sounding task is actually quite difficult. If you can't feel anything, touch a few different objects: your shirt, your head, a chair. Describe *in words* the sensations you feel. Try:

Temperature words (hot, cold, lukewarm, room temperature, absolute zero)
Texture words (smooth, rough, nubby, scratchy, silky, mushy)
Shape words (sharp, rounded, angular, pointy, cylindrical)
Discomfort words (achy, itchy, tired, sore, raw, cramped)

Right now, my hands and feet are feeling: _____

_____

_____

_____

_____

_____

_____

3. *Allow your attention to travel up your arms and legs, through your torso and head. Describe, in words, the physical feelings you observe in your body as a whole.*

This may take a while, and you might feel different things in different parts of your body. Describe all of them. For example, if I do this right now, I notice that my head feels groggy, my neck and shoulders are extremely tight, and I have a slightly nauseated feeling in the pit of my stomach. I'm warm, but not uncomfortably so. Other than that, I feel kind of floppy and relaxed.

Your natural tendency may be to screen out much of the discomfort you feel, or to focus grimly on pain without noticing the good feelings. Allowing both good and bad sensations into consciousness, without resistance, is crucial to staying lean.

Right now, my body as a whole is feeling: _____

_____

_____

_____

_____

_____

_____

_____

4. *Remaining relaxed, describe what you are feeling emotionally. If you can't tell, return your attention to the least comfortable part of your body. Breathe into the discomfort. Allow it to get bigger. Continue this until you sense the emotion connected to the discomfort (there will be one). Describe that emotion in words.*

If I focus on the sensation in my neck and shoulders (currently the part of my body that is least comfortable), I feel . . . wait a second, it's coming to me . . . give it time . . . huh. Frustration, almost mild anger, because I have to go to a dentist appointment in half an hour, and I'd rather keep writing. I didn't know I was feeling frustration until this minute, but there it is.

By the way, if you're like my heaviest clients, you may be thinking that this is touchy-feely pop-psych New Age folderol way beneath your intelligence, and that you'll just skip over this particular exercise. If so, I'll tell you what emotion you're feeling: fear.

Emotion terrifies your computer mind, and if you habitually resist acknowledging painful emotions, you've got a mother load of unfelt feelings bottled up. Notice that you're not *creating* these feelings by paying attention to them. You're just tapping the powder keg you carry around all the time. As you become aware of your emotional state, you may cry, shake, scream, yell, pound your tiny royal fists. Too damn bad. If you want to lose weight, you'll do this step.

Right now, emotionally, I am feeling: _____

_____

_____

_____

_____

_____

_____

_____

_____

5. *Breathe deeply, relax, and notice that on a purely physical level, you're not hungry.*

You may have just connected with terrible sadness over bygone circumstances, such as the premature death of your pet goat, or the excessive longevity of your in-laws. In response to these deep, difficult, painful experiences, I would say to you—and I mean this sincerely: Yeah, yeah, whatever.

Does this shock you? I care very much about your emotions, but I also want you to know that having them doesn't necessarily mean you have to eat. There are other ways to find comfort. At this stage in the process of becoming a thin person, it's only necessary to disentangle the sensations of emotional pain and genuine physical hunger. If you want to eat anyway, just sit with that urge for the 10 minutes it takes to do this exercise. After that, you can eat anything you want.

This may take some time if you're a slow learner like me. I have three degrees from Harvard, have studied creature-talk for decades, and it still takes me at least a minute of focused attention to know whether or not I'm physically hungry. The more time you've spent totally identified with your mind, the more difficult it can be to "hear" what your body is saying. Keep paying attention until you can give your hunger level a score between 0 and 10. Zero means you're feeling no hunger at all, and 10 meaning you're starving. Try it:

Right now, my hunger score is:										
0	1	2	3	4	5	6	7	8	9	10
Not hungry							Ravenous			

Repeat this exercise at least three times a day for 4 days, as you're getting dressed in the morning, during a break or while doing mindless labor in the middle of the day, and when you go to bed at night. Notice the different sensations in your gut under different conditions. Repeat this 4-day win until you can name your hunger score, and differentiate it from an emotion-based eating urge, under any circumstances. Then feel free to move on. You've just mastered a forefield skill—one day you'll want to tap every day to stay tuned in to your creative body.

"Sensation-Interpretation" 4-Day Win

Ridiculously Easy Daily Goal: _Each day for the next 4 days, I'll notice what I'm feeling physically and emotionally. I'll rate my hunger level from 0 to 10 at least three times a day._ _____

Small Daily Reward: _____

_____

Slightly Larger 4-Day Reward: _____

_____

	Dates of My Current 4-Day Win	**Check Off Completed Days Here**
Day 1:	_____ / ____ / _____	_____
Day 2:	_____ / ____ / _____	_____
Day 3:	_____ / ____ / _____	_____
Day 4:	_____ / ____ / _____	_____

If you're already on a weight-loss regimen, remember that the 4-day win will enhance it, not conflict with it. If you know what to do, this program will help you do what you know. Feel free to stay on any weight-loss program while you learn 4-day win skills!

CHAPTER 9

THINKING ABOUT THINKING ABOUT IT

When my youngest child, Elizabeth, was just starting high school, packing her course load with advanced placement classes, I asked her if she'd thought about a college she might one day like to attend.

"Yes I have," she said, firmly. "I want to go someplace that doesn't have bugs. Especially mosquitoes. I hate mosquitoes."

"But . . . " I said, "what about academic specialties? Social life? Job placement?"

Lizzy tensed visibly. "Just no bugs," she said. "That's all I really care about."

My impulse was to push my own agenda, but having observed just how well this worked with my older kids (not), I backed off. Lizzy was in a scared-creature state of mind, focused entirely on biting insects. Pushing her to think otherwise would only have created a polar-bear effect. So I left Lizzy's college choice alone for 2 years. At this writing she's starting her junior year in high school, still taking all the hardest classes she can find, so I decided I'd broach the subject again.

"Any thoughts on college?" I said the other day.

She tensed up again. "I'm not sure."

I was just bristling with good advice, which I have learned is a sure sign I should keep my damn mouth shut. After years as a life coach, I can attest that accepting people as they are is the first thing necessary for positive change to occur.

"I know I have to start thinking about it," said Lizzy.

"Not today, you don't," I said, very much wanting her to think about it. "Today, you don't have to think at all."

There was a long pause. Then Lizzy said, "Well, I think today I'll *think* about thinking about it."

I stayed silent, but inside I was excessively pleased about this tiny parental join-up. Lizzy's scared-creature self, assured that nothing was trying to push her, had articulated the pre-contemplative state of her college choice, and in so doing, moved beyond it. Thinking that it might be time to think about thinking about something is the sign that pre-contemplation is ending. The second stage in the transtheoretical model, "contemplation," is peeking above the horizon.

So far, you've been learning to take the pressure off your scared-animal self by creating an accepting psychological environment where your computer-mind will listen kindly to your creature-self. Now we'll complete the circuit by giving your animal side access to language. Once it has such access, even your most recalcitrant creature features will begin thinking about thinking about losing weight. Slight as it sounds, that little bit of progress means you're on your way to becoming a low-fat version of your present self.

EXPLANATION: BUSTING INTO THE BICAMERAL BRAIN

I once had the extreme good fortune to teach studio art under the professorial auspices of a brilliant artist and teacher, Will Reimann. Mr. Reimann, as I always knew him, recognized that many of his Ivy League students were overly identified with their logical minds. This was in the 1980s, when psychologists were enthusiastically exploring the differences between the right and left hemispheres of the bicameral human brain. Mr. Reimann knew that in general, most academic subjects require the kind of thought that dominates the left hemisphere of the brain: analysis, categorization, calculation, verbal description. Visual art, on the other hand, requires accessing more of the right hemisphere, where synthesis, connection, and imagination reside.

Mr. Reimann was adept at designing exercises that forced his students to use more of their brains' right hemispheres than usual. For example, they spent their first 3 hours of studio time just signing their names—first the normal way, then backwards, then upside down, then upside down and backwards. (If you think this is easy, try it. As a motor skill, signing upside down and backwards is virtually identical to doing it the usual way. But it will make your brain ache like an 80-year-old laundry lady.) Next, the students would have to draw with both hands at once. The left hemisphere of the brain controls the right hand, and vice-versa, so using both hands simultaneously elicits more overall brain activity. (Left-handers are overrepresented in the visual arts, probably because they use the right hemisphere more than right-handers.)

As I worked with all these exercises, I realized that my non-dominant left hand not only functioned more clumsily than its mirror twin, but also seemed to express a different set of thoughts and emotions—things I recognized dimly, if at all, in my logical, verbal thinking. I found that writing with my nondominant hand was exceptionally useful for determining what my subconscious mind was thinking about food and eating.

The exercise in the last chapter is meant to put your mind on the track to understanding your body's signals. This chapter's exercise encourages your unconscious creature mind to speak to you in the language of your computer-self: words. You're going to have a conversation between your dominant and nondominant hands. You'll start with your dominant hand, which is operated by your computer-self. The basic question you're going to ask your creature-self (over and over in different ways, if necessary) is, "How can I help you feel so good that you won't even want to eat for comfort?" Your nondominant hand will provide the answer. No matter what it says, don't judge or attack. If you think your nondominant hand has written something weird, pretend that you're dealing with the beloved only child of your favorite celebrity—and the celebrity happens to be sitting right there. Only allow your computer-self to respond with encouragement, support, curiosity, and a real desire to better the creature-self's life.

EXERCISE: LET YOUR DOMINANT AND NONDOMINANT HANDS CONVERSE

1. Sit down with a notebook, a writing instrument, and at least 10 minutes of time at your disposal.
2. Draw a vertical line down the center of a blank page, dividing it into two columns. Check out the example on page 69 if you're confused about what this should look like.

3. Using your preferred, dominant hand, write a message at the top of the left-hand column. You're writing a note to the part of you that overeats. Start with a greeting, like "Hey, how are you doing right now?"

4. Switch the pencil or pen to your nondominant hand. Position your writing instrument at the top of the right-hand column, directly across from your first message. Start writing with your nondominant hand, responding to the question from your dominant hand. Don't censor, judge, or control the message. Just let it emerge.

5. Switching back to your preferred hand, write another message in the left column, under "Hey, how are you doing?" I suggest you use the phrase, "What can I do to help you feel so good you won't want to eat?"

6. Switch back to the nondominant hand, and write whatever comes up in response.

7. Continue to go back and forth, using your dominant hand to non-judgmentally ask how you (that is, your computer-self) can make your nondominant hand (that is, your creature-self) comfortable, happy, and relaxed. No matter what emerges, do not judge or condemn your creature self. Just keep offering to help.

8. When your nondominant hand writes a message signifying willingness to cooperate, wish it well and conclude your session. This sometimes takes up to 10 minutes, but you may find that you come to an agreement between your computer-self and you creature-self almost immediately. The more time you've spent dieting, the longer it will take.

EXAMPLE OF BICAMERAL BRAIN CONVERSATION

I've been doing this exercise periodically for years. When I began, my nondominant side was very, very unhappy with the dominant side, but this changed over the years until we're on rather good terms. Here are a couple of examples:

My First Creature-Computer Dialogue Session: Circa May 1998

COMPUTER (DOMINANT HAND)	CREATURE (NONDOMINANT HAND)
Hey, how you doing?	$%^& you.
What can I do for you?	You can %^&* $%
I know I've ignored you for years, but I'm going to make it up to you.	Oh, right. &*(# Atkins &*^(#@$^ grapefruit %^&* $%^& !@#$ Pritikin #^$^.
What would you think of eating moderate amounts of healthy food today?	&% cake Pop Tarts onion dip baklava buffalo wings ^&%(# (^& cake mix Cheez Whiz Key Lime pie. NOW!

My (Approximately) 2787th Session: June 2006

COMPUTER (DOMINANT HAND)	CREATURE (NONDOMINANT HAND)
Hey, how you doing?	Not bad. You?
I'm fine. Listen, how would you feel about eating nothing but texturized vegetable protein today?	YEUCH, I hate that stuff. I think aliens invented it to feed to people they abduct.
Yes, I know, but I'm doing an experiment for this book I'm writing.	Oh, all right. Can I paint? A landscape with a lot of yellow? I want yellow.
Well, I really have to write...	If you won't let me paint, I'll eat Twizzlers all day. Plus, I'll freeze your brain so you CAN'T write.
Okay, okay! I have to phone a client later. You can paint the whole time.	You've got yourself a deal.

MOVING INTO CONTEMPLATION

As you can see, my creature-self often trades on its power to insist that I do its favorite things. The more relaxed and practiced you get with this exercise, the more you'll find that odd, non-food-related ideas will emerge from your nondominant hand. Remember what I said in Chapter 1, about 4-day wins making you happier, as well as leaner? As you connect with the creature side of your nature through this exercise, you'll begin to see glimmers of new directions you'll take in your life as a whole. Virtually every client I've worked with on weight has come up with ideas, activities, goals, and aspirations they'd denied, ignored, or abandoned during their chubby years.

This is a subject we'll cover much more thoroughly as we move through the transtheoretical model of change. For now, the point is that if you want to control your own diet and exercise patterns, it helps to give your creature-self the means and opportunity to speak to you in writing. Once you've learned to interpret its language (the language of feelings) and it begins speaking in yours (the language of words), you're ready to move out of Stage 1, pre-contemplation, and into Stage 2, comtemplative. And that means, oh gentle reader, that it's time for you to learn The Most Important Weight-Loss Skill in the History of the Universe.

"Nondominant Hand" 4-Day Win

Ridiculously Easy Daily Goal: _Each day for the next 4 days, I'll write a conversation between my dominant and nondominant hands. With my dominant hand, I'll ask for cooperation in eating healthily. I'll allow my nondominant hand to respond in any way it wants._ _____

Small Daily Reward: _____

_____

Slightly Larger 4-Day Reward: _____

_____

	Dates of My **Current 4-Day Win**	**Check Off** **Completed Days Here**
Day 1:	_____ / ____ / _____	_____
Day 2:	_____ / ____ / _____	_____
Day 3:	_____ / ____ / _____	_____
Day 4:	_____ / ____ / _____	_____

If you're already on a weight-loss regimen, remember that the 4-day win will enhance it, not conflict with it. If you know what to do, this program will help you do what you know. Feel free to stay on any weight-loss program while you learn 4-day win skills!

STAGE
2

CONTEMPLATION

Hallo! If you're on the Jump-Start plan, you've read this chapter. Glance over it again, to see how it fits into the 4-day win program as a whole. Continue!

CHAPTER 10

THE MOST IMPORTANT WEIGHT-LOSS SKILL IN THE HISTORY OF THE UNIVERSE

From where I'm sitting, the most promising weight-loss strategies aren't new diets or more insistent exhortations to control ourselves, but the implications of new research on brain function, which shows that the command center in our heads can basically be changed by experience—a phenomenon called neuroplasticity. Where I'm sitting, by the way, is in an office chair at a clinic that offers "brain mapping." The folks who work here wire up people's heads, plug them into computers, and collect all sorts of real-time data about the electrical activity generated by their brains.

So far, my brain-mapping results indicate that I have serious attention deficit disorder, but compensate for it with astronomical anxiety. This explains why my day-to-day train of thought goes like this: *Look! A shiny object! What's that doing in the—oh my God, I forgot to [call the plumber/ e-mail my editor/feed the children/dress myself]! I'd better get that done right awa—Hey, look! A shiny object!"*

Fortunately, neuroscience has recently determined that I can deliberately alter the way my brain works. So far, I've spent more than 10 hours in this chair, watching a line on the monitor that shows how vigorously my brain is producing beta waves, which are associated with anxiety. I'm "training down" my anxiety by doing whatever it takes to make that line drop. The process is hard to describe. I've found that the line goes down when I create a certain warm pressure in the middle of my head, but I can't tell you how I do it. Even so, I think it's working; I feel quite drunk with calm as my brain makes the adjustment. My anxiety has been much lower lately, in every situation. It feels fabulous. Though I have no earthly idea where I left my children.

My point is that we don't need to be doomed to corpulence just because our brains evolved to resist weight loss. We can out-think our own biology. However, as we've seen, simply imposing conscious will on our bodies won't work. It requires a new skill, one that's completely unfamiliar to most people and feels so subtle that we overlook its power: watching ourselves think, without getting caught up in our thoughts. And it's one we can acquire without leaving our own living room chairs.

EXPLANATION: RETROFITTING YOUR BRAIN

Jeffrey Schwartz, MD, is a psychiatrist who treats patients with obsessive-compulsive disorder (OCD). People who have OCD feel compelled to repeat behaviors like handwashing, even when they know it's excessive. If they don't wash their hands when the urge hits them, they feel incredibly high anxiety. Many psychologists use the classic diet advisor's "just stop it!" approach to treat these patients, forcing them to do things like hold dog feces without washing their hands. Surprise, surprise, this tends to be counterproductive. Most patients can defy their anxiety in the short term, but in the long run, they often backlash and become more compulsive than ever.

To Dr. Schwartz, this white-knuckle approach made no sense. He knew that on brain scans, people with OCD show unusually high activity in the part of the brain that triggers fear reactions. He could take pictures of this, MRI images that showed an electrically hyperactive spot in his patients' frontal lobes. He gave his patients these pictures of their brains overreacting. When the handwashing urge hit, Dr. Schwartz had them look at the MRIs and tell themselves, "It feels like I should wash my hand, but really, this is just an electrical impulse in my brain." Then they'd do something they enjoyed—Dr. Schwartz mentions gardening, though I prefer making crank telephone calls to elected officials—for 15 minutes.

At first, some of Dr. Schwartz's patients had to repeat this, but after a maximum of two 15-minute sessions, the urge to wash their hands had subsided. The longer they persisted with this exercise, the shorter the duration of their urges. Finally, the handwashing anxiety would stop. At that point, Dr. Schwartz took more MRI images—and found that the structure of his patients' "abnormal" brains had changed. Their brains were now structurally normal.

I believe (and early research suggests) that overeating is often a self-calming compulsion similar to OCD. When a handwasher gets psychologically stressed, say by the unsettling illness of a pet goldfish, that person's first reaction may be to crank up the faucets. For a compulsive eater like me, Mr. Fin's declining health would lead straight to a pound cake. Being barred from eating used to cause me enormous discomfort—not physical hunger, but the same freakout experienced by handwashers who can't get to the sink. For anyone who's ever been calorie-deprived by dieting, actual hunger can be terrifying. We can't overcome this by going on stricter diets, any more than an obsessive-compulsive handwasher can achieve normalcy by clutching dog poo.

The exercise you're about to learn will help you respond effectively to stress without having to eat anything. I believe that, in a process similar to the one Dr. Schwartz observed in his patients, *practicing the exercise repeatedly may alter the physical structure of your brain, so that you no longer feel any need to eat when you aren't hungry.* It's so subtle you may at first underestimate its power, but if it's the only thing you learn from this book, practicing it regularly can stop you from overeating.

This exercise will quietly remove you from Stage 1, the "pre-contemplative" state where most dieters are stuck, unconsciously, for most of their lives. Various versions of this practice exist in every culture that has a tradition of "contemplation." Contemplatives are people who stand back a step from the usual grimy struggle of human activity, seeing and thinking with unusual clarity. They're also the members of any given culture who can do extraordinary things, like staying calm in disasters, providing wisdom in times of crisis, accessing mystical states, and imagining Donald Trump with normal hair. You don't have to believe in shamanism to take advantage of the contemplatives' way of being. It can happen anytime you change your behavior by emerging from Stage 1, Pre-contemplation to Stage 2, Contemplation. This next lesson will teach you to become the kind of contemplative I call the Watcher.

EXERCISE: THE WATCHER, THE DICTATOR, AND THE WILD CHILD

In Chapter 6, I asked you to recall the set of controlling, bitter thoughts with which your mind tries to lash you to various weight-loss regimens. These words, like all verbal thinking, are produced by the computer-self. You saw how your creature-self reacts, by panicking and breaking the rules. In this chapter, we'll picture these rule-making and rule-breaking parts of you as humans. Tiny humans. We'll call them the Dictator and the Wild Child.

The instructions below may feel odd, but I want you to follow them anyway because of the way they affect your brain. First, hold out your right hand, palm up. Imagine a 2-inch-tall version of yourself in a military uniform, with a whip in one hand and a gun in the other, stomping around in your palm, shrieking deeply personal insults and commanding you to lose weight. This is the Dictator. Now hold up your left palm (you may have to put down this book for a minute) and picture your Wild Child there: 2 inches tall, dressed in skins and bark, covered with scars, waiting for an opportunity to escape or subvert the Dictator's brutal control. Watch until you can see them both clearly in your mind's eye.

Now, while watching these two mini-you's, I want you to see that as dysfunctional as they may be, both of them are essentially good. The Dictator wants you to be healthy and beautiful. It gets frantic about your weight for the same reason you might freak out if you saw a beloved pet wandering into traffic. It screams and yells, pens you in or drags you around—anything to keep you from a horrible fat fate. On the other hand, the Wild Child is the part of you that evolved to avoid starvation and captivity. It panics when the Dictator berates, shames, and tries to control it. It knows the Dictator is planning to starve it. So it's not surprising that the instant the Dictator is weakened by stress, hunger, or environmental chaos, the Wild Child leaps into action and eats like a junkyard dog.

Think through the well-meaning motivations of both your Dictator and your Wild Child, until you really understand that within their limited perspectives they're doing their very best. Then offer them both kindness. One useful method is to silently repeat these phrases from the classic "loving-kindness" meditation: *"May you be well. May you be happy. May you be free from suffering."* It may help to set the book aside again and close your eyes. Continue offering these good wishes while visualizing both the Wild Child and the Dictator until you genuinely mean it, until you can feel compassion toward both sides of yourself. When you get there, consider the following question.

Who are you?

The only reason you can "see" and offer kindness to both Dictator and the Wild Child is that you're not either one of them. You've moved into a third realm of consciousness, which resides, literally, in a different part of your brain. Call it the Watcher.

This is a subtle transition. You may feel it as a slight sense of loosening and relief, the psychological equivalent of taking off a tight, itchy piece of clothing. Or it might feel revolutionary, an epiphany that changes you permanently the first time you feel it. I've seen many people who do this exercise begin to cry—and these are individuals who've been through 17 kinds of hell without shedding a tear. Often, I get a specific sensation when someone near me moves into the Watcher-self. It's as though an enormous, powerful, invisible creature has slipped soundlessly into the room and settled itself against the wall. It raises every hair on my body.

You may not feel this at first, or it may be so inconspicuous that you don't even notice it. Just persist with the exercise, offering the Dictator and Wild Child best wishes for at least a full minute at a time (it often takes about 50 seconds for a beginner). When you can clearly imagine both sides of your dieting self, without identifying completely with either of them, consider another question:

Holding this mental position, how do you feel about food?

While both the Dictator and Wild Child make you want to overeat, your Watcher self is not nearly as compulsive. It doesn't feel either rigidly controlled or totally out-of-control. In fact, according to some medical psychologists, it's physiologically impossible for your mind to stay locked in a war of control when you're engaging its ability to generate compassion and appreciation. It is a place of great inner peace. Since it's also the only mindset from which you can make yourself an effortlessly lean person, I call it "the place of Thinner Peace." True, this is a roll-your-eyes pun, but it gives me a memorable label for a distinct inner sensation. I know from brain mapping that this is literally the feeling of my brain releasing anxiety.

THINNER PEACE: KEYS TO
THE KINGDOM

I can't stress this strongly enough: Learning to access the place of Thinner Peace is *the most important weight-loss skill in the history of the universe*, and it will enable you to stay on any weight-loss regimen. And now that you've learned about and practiced the pre-contemplative and contemplative skills discussed in the preceding chapters, you're ready to integrate this crucial skill into your life.

Almost all of us assume there's only one way to lose weight: by willpower, by white-knuckle resistance, by forcing the body with an aggressive, adversarial, disciplinarian mind. This can be achieved *sometimes*, though not often. Maintaining it long-term? I don't think that can be done. I've seen numerous clients deploy incredible discipline, using their Dictator selves to trap, dominate, and starve their Wild Child selves. Losing weight this way is as draining as keeping a violent criminal pinned to the floor with sheer force. But even if you manage to do it, you can't hold your own Wild Child in a hammerlock for the rest of your life. The minute you get tired, distracted, or sick, the Dictator loses control, and the Wild Child goes into a feeding frenzy.

That's the whole reason I wrote this book. Simply going on a diet program, without changing your mental set, causes backlash and weight gain. *This is an inevitable reality, based on the way our brains and bodies are designed.* But if you use 4-day win techniques to become a Watcher and bring yourself to Thinner Peace, your brain changes, as well as your body. Weight loss happens without backlash or resistance.

The deceptively quiet power of this brain-shifting strategy has made it a favorite of contemplatives in many places, throughout time. Stepping back from the Dictator and the Wild Child and becoming the Watcher is like thinking you've been stuck on a railroad track, able to move only backward and forward, and discovering that you had the capacity to fly all along. Even if this initially only feels like a tiny hop off the tracks, it can be the beginning of a whole new life. Becoming a Watcher is a forefield skill, one you'll want to use daily, or even several times a day, once you master it. To begin, try this 4-day win:

"Becoming the Watcher"
4-Day Win

Ridiculously Easy Daily Goal: *Each day for the next 4 days, I'll visualize my Dictator and Wild Child sides, one in each hand. I'll offer them compassion until I can feel that I am not either one of them.*

Small Daily Reward: _____

_____

Slightly Larger 4-Day Reward: _____

_____

	Dates of My Current 4-Day Win	**Check Off Completed Days Here**
Day 1:	____/____/____	_____
Day 2:	____/____/____	_____
Day 3:	____/____/____	_____
Day 4:	____/____/____	_____

If you're already on a weight-loss regimen, remember that the 4-day win will enhance it, not conflict with it. If you know what to do, this program will help you do what you know. Feel free to stay on any weight-loss program while you learn 4-day win skills!

CHAPTER 11

LEARN
TO RETURN
TO THE PLACE
OF THINNER
PEACE

A common crime in certain areas, such as third-world slums, the musical *Rent*, and my teenagers' bedrooms, is something called "theft of electricity." Electricity thieves are people who can't afford to pay utility bills, so they jury-rig public wires to connect to their personal appliances. Well, your brain is basically an organic electrical appliance. When you think, electricity passes between neurons in various parts of your brain, creating all sorts of sensations and operations. When you connect with the Thinner Peace aspect of your consciousness, you "steal" electricity from the parts of your brain that create destructive thinking and overeating. It diverts this energy into the areas of the brain that relieve compulsions and produce a sensation of bliss. Unfortunately, those same areas are busy trying to steal electricity from the calming parts of your brain. It's a Con Edison battle royale.

Throughout human history, full-time contemplatives like monks, shamans, and gurus have made the process of accessing the brain's place of peace the core of their daily work. To master re-channeling their own brain waves, they often retreat from society into the wilderness, where they'll encounter minimum distraction. But you probably don't awaken every morning to watch in silence as the sun rises over the Himalayas. Instead, you drag yourself out of bed after too little sleep, pull on uncomfortable clothes, rush the kids to school, and jostle your way through gridlocked traffic to work for a boss so infuriating he would make Jesus long for Xanax. Surrounding you, everpresent, is a veritable ocean of cheap, fattening food. It's no wonder you break your healthy-eating vows. Something's gotta give.

The 4-day win we'll explore in this chapter can help you put yourself in the brain-state of the peaceful, compassionate Watcher even under the adverse conditions of your daily life. These are techniques by which you "learn to return" when you've strayed into anxiety, anger, or other conditions that may trigger overeating. If you've done all the exercises in this book, so far, you've learned to create small islands in time and space where you can feel safe, become very relaxed, move your consciousness into relative tranquility, and feel less compelled to eat. Now I want you to expand that skill set, so that you can begin to create this chain of events under more and more challenging conditions.

EXPLANATION: BENEVOLENT BRAIN BANDITRY

The fear-based parts of your brain are many, varied, and ancient. Alarm responses, particularly the fear of attack and starvation, improve any animal's chances of survival in a wild state where hunger and being hunted are major threats. As a result, evolution has selected for them very powerfully. These responses were present in reptiles long before the first human stomped the earth, so scientists refer to the primitive brain structure that triggers flight-or-fight responses (even in humans) as the "reptilian brain."

The ability to let go of all fear and surrender to a state of boundaryless bliss, on the other hand, is a much rarer brain state. While virtually everyone suffers and feels fear, many people live and die without ever experiencing inner peace. Being able to eat or stop eating by choice and without any anxiety means gently detaching yourself from negative reactions to all stress, including the fear of physical hunger.

This virtually never happens by chance. Given our hard-wiring, the likelihood that we'll naturally become fearful and panicky under pressure is right around 100 percent. The likelihood of using either nachos or chocolate to deal with this, for a standard American at room temperature, is considerably higher than that. Telling ourselves to stop eating *stop eating STOP EATING, DAMMIT,* only creates a feedback screech, which, according to numeric calculations I am making up specifically for this paragraph, more than doubles this risk.

Fortunately (and this I am *not* making up), advanced contemplatives have always taught that an enlightened mind is not a mind totally unacquainted with fear, conflict, or self-destructive behavior, but one in which fear, conflict, and self-destructive behavior are greeted with the indefatigable willingness to return to a peaceful state. For thousands of years, these gifted contemplatives have learned and taught methodologies for diverting the electrical energy of the brain from fear to calm. Using these methods is like setting Robin Hood loose in your head, to steal electricity from corrupt, violent powers and redistribute it to the aspects of your mind that will use it for benevolent purposes. Here are three techniques I've found especially useful for returning to the mental state that facilitates weight loss.

EXERCISE: RETURN, RETURN, RETURN

TECHNIQUE #1: THREE BREATHS

This advice is so ubiquitous that I actually find it annoying. Every ancient text on mystical bliss, every yoga teacher in the world, every newspaper article on stress reduction will tell you that deep, regular breathing is the starting point for stilling inner turmoil. I know, I know, you've heard that a gazillion times. That's because it works.

According to psychologist Tom Kenyon, the core survival function of breathing is so wired into the brain that every time our moods or environment change, it subtly (or dramatically) changes our breath pattern. The interesting thing is that this also works in reverse: if you deliberately breathe in a way that's characteristically associated with an emotion (fear, sexual arousal, anger, excitement, joy, etc.) you'll activate the same part of your brain that creates the emotional energy, and experience the emotion connected to each specific breathing pattern. (You may want to experiment with this: "fake" a feeling, exaggerate the breathing pattern that emerges, and watch emotions arise. The better you are at mimicking the breathing pattern, the stronger the mood effect will be.)

I've met Buddhist monks who spent *years* just paying attention to their breathing, and they seem like very happy people with minimal body fat. But their single-minded persistence is way, way beyond me. I prefer an exercise for us nonmonk mortals, which is called "the three breaths." When you find yourself stressed, tense, and veering toward anxiety eating, take a time-out for just three breaths. Long, deep breaths. You can panic again as soon as the third exhalation has left your lungs. But you probably won't. It's amazing how much your mind and body will calm down if you just completely fill and empty your lung three times. Try this the next time (in fact, every time) you feel emotionally upset, physically numb, or unhappy about your weight. Move into the Watcher identity by offering yourself compassionate wishes ("May you be well, may you be happy, may you be free from suffering") until you feel a physical relaxation response.

Here's a useful trick for making it easier to recapture the Watcher's peaceful frame of mind: once you feel relaxed, squeeze the pinky finger of your left hand in your right fist. This inconspicuous behavior will associate a concrete, physical action with the mental condition of noncompulsive calm. (Practitioners of neuro-linguistic programming call it "stacking.") You know how old memories come flooding back when you taste tea and a Madeleine (if you happen to be Proust) or revisit your childhood home? This is called "state-dependent memory." It's so powerful that when diabetics are given insulin injections in a room painted with a big yellow zigzag, and then later go into that room without having an injection, their insulin levels rise sharply, exactly as if they'd been given a shot. Squeezing your pinky finger at times when you're feeling peaceful creates a state-dependent association between the relaxation response and a deliberate physical sensation. The next time you feel anxious, simply squeezing your pinky can help trigger the same relaxation response.

TECHNIQUE #2: TREASURE CHESTS

To get this exercise started, you'll need another 5 to 10 minutes of quiet time. After that, you can use the technique almost instantaneously when the need arises. Begin by picturing the inside of your head as a roundish room. You're standing in the center, and around the periphery, you see several large wooden chests, like pirate's treasure chests. Each crate contains an assortment of memories categorized by emotional similarity (by the way, the brain really does store your memories this way; when neurosurgeons stimulate adjacent brain areas, patients have vivid memories that are related by topic—though topics are selected differently by each individual).

Now, some of the brain-boxes in the round room have skulls and crossbones painted on them. They hold memories of fear, lack, humiliation, abuse, all the dark and gloomy things you've experienced. These memories are like objects made of razor wire, broken glass, and acid. If you "pick them up," by brooding on them or grasping them tightly, you will feel enormous pain. You'll get more and more depressed, enraged, or anxious the more tightly you grip them.

There are, however, other boxes in your brain with more cheerful labels. There's your box of puppy memories, your sunny vacation reminiscences, your recollection of all those happy hours applying watercolor paint to chicken bones. (I actually did this a lot as a child. We didn't have a television.) Everywhere you look are treasures: memories of winning an award, quitting that awful job, holding your brand new baby, going for a sunrise swim in the ocean and being joined by a pod of dolphins.

The treasure chest technique simply requires that you temporarily put down hurtful brain-toys, and pick up your treasures instead. This doesn't mean you need to stop honoring your history of trauma or loss, it just means you have the option of focusing on other things when you want to. Visualize going over to a chest that says, "Hiking" or "Laughter" or "Beauty" or "Times I Made Things Explode." Open the box. Take out a memory. Recall it very vividly. Then go back to another treasure chest and find another priceless moment. Write down 10 of them. Then read over your list, relive the experiences, and squeeze your pinky finger to anchor the sensation.

Ten "Treasure-Chest" Memories

1. _____

2. _____

3. _____

4. _____

5. _____

6. _____

7. _____

8. _____

9. _____

10. _____

TECHNIQUE #3: THICK DESCRIPTION

Social scientists who study unfamiliar cultures are trained to use a technique called "thick description." This means noting every possible physical detail of a situation without judgment. An anthropologist might write: "We proceeded into the cave, where the women of the tribe had lit a large fire, in which they were heating softball-size stones. The cave was approximately the size of a convenience store, but lacked Slurpee drink dispensers. The floor was dusty and had small bones and feathers strewn here and there. The walls were coated with a thick layer of smoke. The firepit was approximately 4 feet in diameter. The chief informed me it was used for cooking chickens, pigs, anthropologists, deer, blah blah blah."

This technique, though useful, can be incredibly boring—unless it's a description of your own best memories. Right now, choose one of the memories you found in your "treasure chest," and write (or silently narrate) a "thick description" of that memory. "It was April in Paris, and the air smelled of rain and apple blossoms. I sat at a tiny café table made of cold wrought iron. The people across from me were arguing about Sartre. Their voices were querulous and nasal." Etc., etc. The more detailed and sensory your description (think of smells, sounds, tastes, and touch as well as sights), the more this process of thick description will move you away from the anxiety-ridden, overeating part of your brain, and into the purely perceptive areas that connect you to Thinner Peace.

Thick Description of a Wonderful Memory

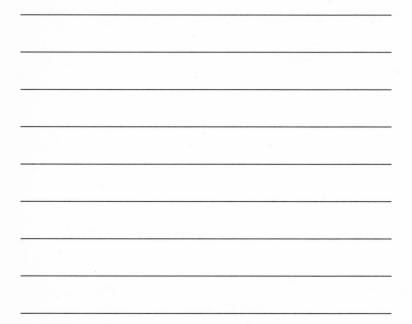

Read over your "thick description" while you squeeze your pinky finger, attaching ever more pleasant associations to that physical action and sensation. For your next 4-day win, spend 10 relaxed minutes a day linking up with pleasurable memories. Do this while you're stopped at a traffic light, waiting at the bank, or lying in bed before falling asleep. Get accustomed to playing with moments of pleasure and delight, instead of engaging with bitterness and fear, when your brain is idling. Once you've learned to return to that April-in-Paris café, falling in love, or holding your new baby as the dolphins play around you, you're ready to start the part of "contemplation" that will change the way you eat.

"Learn to Return" 4-Day Win

Ridiculously Easy Daily Goal: _Each day for the next 4 days, I'll spend 10_

minutes deliberately replaying positive memories in great detail, while breathing

deeply and squeezing my left pinky finger in my right hand.

Small Daily Reward: _____

_____

Slightly Larger 4-Day Reward: _____

_____

	Dates of My Current 4-Day Win	Check Off Completed Days Here
Day 1:	____/____/____	_____
Day 2:	____/____/____	_____
Day 3:	____/____/____	_____
Day 4:	____/____/____	_____

If you're already on a weight-loss regimen, remember that the 4-day win will enhance it, not conflict with it. If you know what to do, this program will help you do what you know. Feel free to stay on any weight-loss program while you learn 4-day win skills!

CHAPTER 12

HOW TO STOP EATING WHEN YOU CAN'T STOP EATING

Dave is one of the strongest, toughest, most successful people I know. A nationally prominent trial attorney, he's in his late 30s, athletic, drop-dead handsome, wealthy, and is loved by his devoted family. He's also committing suicide. Weapon of choice: doughnuts.

I don't just mean Dave is munching his way to ordinary love handles and high cholesterol. He has medical conditions that make unhealthy eating especially dangerous for him: type II diabetes and celiac disease (which makes him unable to tolerate the gluten found in wheat and other grains). For you, a doughnut may be an indulgence; for Dave, it's literally poison. His doctors have told him his life is in imminent danger if he doesn't stick to a healthy, sugar-free, gluten-free menu. Yet the last time I spoke to him, he'd just been to a wedding where he stood by the buffet line and ate pastries one after another, without even taking them to his table.

Again, people who think Dave's problem is lack of willpower are utterly wrong. The force imposed by the inner Dictator is equaled by the backlash of the Wild Child; Dave eats countless doughnuts precisely because he's very strong-willed and very scared of what will happen to him if he eats doughnuts. He's gained almost 75 pounds since his diagnosis, and no coercive force—no doctor's warning, no symptoms of illness, no amount of raw fear—is going to stop this. The only way for Dave to save his life is to develop a habit of becoming his peaceful Watcher self even in conditions of outright warfare, such as standing at a buffet table.

The same may be true of you. Filling your fridge with lettuce and fish may keep you on the dietary straight and narrow part of the time, but to the extent that you're anxious about your weight and struggling against the desire to gorge on wickedly fattening food, you live on a battlefield. When the combat is at its height, when the world seems determined to lob missiles of buttery, sugary, oily junk food directly in your path, you may have very little ability to control your eating, no matter how well-informed and well-meaning you may be.

EXPLANATION: THE WARP SPASM

Dave happens to be of Irish heritage. The ancient Irish were rowdy, competitive warriors who laughed at danger and had no tolerance for cringing or moping. To this day, Irish Americans like Dave enjoy gathering in pubs where they occupy themselves by competing at darts, telling hilarious tales, and refusing to show weakness. Now, according to Irish legend, some warriors were so fightin' fit that during a battle, they'd be taken over by something called the "warp spasm." When the warp spasm hit, the fighter achieved superhuman strength and ferocity. Here's how one account describes the warp spasm of the famous warrior Cúchulain:

> This frenzy caused him to turn about in his skin; his sinews bulged with knots the size of a baby's head; a poisonous black mist rose above his head; and he snapped his jaw shut with enough force to kill a lion, showering sparks. In this fearsome state he could not tell friend from foe, killing in front and behind alike.

Does this sound familiar to you? If you've ever had a hard-core eating binge, it might. Dave certainly identifies with it, because it's a lot like what happened to him at that wedding. Extreme overeating is basically a warp spasm, a violent tantrum thrown by the deprived or captive Wild Child in our brains. When it hits, rational thinking goes out the window. Dave's doctors said he should be more logical about his eating choices. They might as well have told him to stop a tidal wave by insisting that it apply for a beach permit.

The warp spasm is driven by fear. Every time he sees forbidden food, a terrifying battle ensues in Dave's mind. He's afraid of what will happen if he eats it, and he's afraid he won't be able *not* to eat it. Being a big strong Irish man, Dave doesn't experience either fear consciously. He just locks eyes with the nearest pastry tray and goes into a warp spasm, "snapping his jaws shut with enough force to kill a lion" on pastry after pastry. He's in a kind of wild trance, unaware of any feelings, having no logical thoughts at all.

THE PSYCHOLOGY OF THE BINGE TRANCE

In any situation where our brains perceive extreme threat, the neocortex (the most recently evolved layer of the brain, which performs logical calculation) may be "hijacked" by the deeper, more primitive reptilian layer. If you've ever been in a car crash where time seemed to stop, slow down, or speed up, it's because your neocortex is the part of your brain that tracks time. When it's been "hijacked," you don't perceive time the way you usually do. You're in a fight or flight response, your body is pumping out stress hormones, and your attention riveted on survival behaviors like escaping, hording, and packing on fat against the threat of famine.

Once this happens to Dave, there's no turning back. He could take a bullet and keep swallowing. So he eats himself sick, then retreats to his bedroom and lies in the dark, filled with food, nausea, torpor, shame, self-hatred, and fear. He chastises himself brutally for being weak—which intensifies his inner war, making him more likely to binge again. Dave's loved ones and doctors encourage his self-hatred, thinking it will make him stop bingeing, when the opposite is true. *The only way to get out of this suicidal pattern is to leave the battlefield by going to the Watcher's place of peace.*

EXERCISE: FINDING THINNER PEACE IN WARTIME

If you've tried to diet before, you've probably had some version of a bingeing warp spasm, though not, I hope, one as extreme as Dave's. The bad news is that the more deeply you've sunk into this pattern, the more time it may take for your particular weight war to end. The good news is that *you can step off the battlefield any time.* You do this by aligning yourself with the Watcher part of your brain, then observing the conflict from a kind, detached distance. The more time you spend observing the battles, the less energy the war will have, and the sooner it will end. Strange but true: the brain that observes itself, changes itself.

A wonderful opportunity to practice this skill occurs in the exhausted torpor after you've had yourself a warp spasm. Use the following exercise when the spasm is over, at the point where you'd usually descend into self-loathing. If you do this exercise consistently, you'll regain a sense of stability, safety, and noncompulsiveness sooner and sooner after every binge. One day, you'll be able to access your Watcher self while the binge is actually happening. This is an odd sensation, like screaming in fear at a Halloween "haunted house" while knowing all the time that you're perfectly safe. You'll watch yourself go into the binge trance, hear the Dictator shouting "No! No! Don't eat, you worthless bag of crap!" You'll feel the Wild Child's defiance, its violent enjoyment of the destructive, degrading feeding frenzy. But you'll also feel, at the very same time, that a part of you exists outside this dichotomy. You aren't the Dictator and you aren't the Wild Child, but the calm presence that sees each of them as transitory and ultimately insubstantial. You are the Watcher of this warp spasm, not identified completely with it.

Soon after this occurs, you'll begin to notice your warp spasms just *before* they take over. One day, you'll feel this happening, slip into the identity of the Watcher, and find that the binge trance rises, falls, then disappears within about 30 seconds. You'll literally forget to binge, as though pigging out is a mildly unpleasant but unnecessary task that you just can't motivate yourself to complete. Not long after that, you'll realize that you're far happier when you're in the Watcher state of mind, so you'll stay there most of the time. Persist long enough, and your overeating warp spasms will become mild, occasional, or nonexistent.

Beating the Binge Monster

1. Create a relaxation response as you did in Chapter 5: Get to a safe place; breathe, notice your physical sensations, then emotional ones. Repeat affirmations like "I don't have to do anything right now," until you can accept what you are feeling for this moment. Keep deepening your breathing and acceptance until you feel your muscles relax.

2. Recall a recent occasion when you overate—the more out-of-control, the better for practicing your new self-calming skills. Jot a few words here to remind yourself of the incident (for example, "At Joe's bar mitzvah," or "2 a.m. this morning.")

3. In memory, walk through the experience of the binge. Recall as much as you can about the setting, what you were feeling physically, and how the binge played out. As you remember, notice any changes in your breathing, muscle tension, and body position. You may flinch or get extremely fidgety. *Do not run away or stop the exercise.* Breathe in, exhale, and continue to relax with the memory still in mind.

4. As you watch the memory of your binge, notice what you were feeling emotionally. You may actually re-experience some of the emotions that drove the binge, such as anxiety, anger, sadness, or manic excitement. Watch them without moving. Notice that your Wild Child was trying to heal or express itself by overeating.

5. Now focus on the shame or self-loathing you felt once the eating finally stopped. Listen to the abusive or hopeless things you've said to yourself in this state of remorseful regret. Feel the anxiety that drove your self-accusations. Notice that this is your inner Dictator, and that it is well-meaning but counterproductive. It only makes the Wild Child feel even more misunderstood, abused, and disconsolate.

6. For six full breaths, detach from the Wild Child and the Dictator by picturing both, simultaneously, and offering them kind wishes: "May you be well. May you be happy. May you be free from suffering." Notice that as you identify with the Watcher, your anger at yourself for bingeing, and the fear that you will binge again, become less intense. As you practice this exercise repeatedly, you'll find that the effect can be dramatic, quick, and incredibly calming.

7. Replay the scene of the binge one more time, observing it as the Watcher and offering kindness to your bingeing self the entire time. Continue until you can remain physically relaxed with the memory still in mind. If you can, imagine being in the same situation without eating, using kindness to nourish a state of calm relaxation.

8. Stay in this relaxed state for 5 minutes or as long as you can, whichever arrives first.

Dave had to spend about 20 minutes on this exercise before he was able to replay the memory of the wedding banquet without feeling compulsive, ashamed, anxious, or out of control. But by taking this time, he began the process of walking away from all sorts of dietary battlefields, *before* being overtaken by the warp spasm and developing sinew-knots the size of a baby's head, which has got to be good for his social life. (I'll share more of Dave's story in later chapters.) As you go through your 4-day win on this exercise, you'll connect more and more easily to the part of your brain that is calm, happy, and free from trancelike compulsive eating. Your mind may still be warped, of course—considering it's you we're talking about—but not when it comes to food.

"Beating the Binge Monster" 4-Day Win

Ridiculously Easy Daily Goal: _Each day for the next 4 days, I'll revisit a time I overate or felt out of control of my eating. I'll persist until I can relax throughout the entire memory._

Small Daily Reward: _____

_____

Slightly Larger 4-Day Reward: _____

_____

	Dates of My Current 4-Day Win	Check Off Completed Days Here
Day 1:	___ / ___ / ___	_____
Day 2:	___ / ___ / ___	_____
Day 3:	___ / ___ / ___	_____
Day 4:	___ / ___ / ___	_____

If you're already on a weight-loss regimen, remember that the 4-day win will enhance it, not conflict with it. If you know what to do, this program will help you do what you know. Feel free to stay on any weight-loss program while you learn 4-day win skills!

CHAPTER 13

MAKE LOVE, NOT WAR

LIVING IN THE PLACE OF PEACE

In the early years of the 21st century, a cheerful band of Tibetan lamas graciously allowed researchers at the University of Wisconsin to wire up their shaven heads and peer into their brains. All these lamas had spent many years practicing Tibetan meditation, which involves the compassionate self-observation similar to the exercises you've been learning during your last few 4-day wins. It turned out that the monks had unusual brains; compared to most people, they had more activity in the left prefrontal cortex, a brain region associated with happiness. The longer a monk had been meditating, the larger and more active this part of his brain.

Don't worry, I'm not about to tell you that losing weight requires endless chanting in the flickering light of yak-butter candles. If I tried to do this, I'd freak out and eat every last candle, not to mention some of the yaks, within hours. But research on meditation does indicate that staying in a compassionate mode toward one's self removes brain activity from zones that trigger flight, fight, and frenzied eating. So far in your "contemplation" strategy, you've learned to:

1. Access the peaceful Watcher aspect of your consciousness with focused attention
2. Return to it at random moments throughout the day

3. Trigger it with visualizations and physical sensations
4. Use it to calm yourself in times of dieting crisis.

You've taken a few jaunts away from the weight-loss battlefield, into the demilitarized zone. Now, I'd like you to consider something truly radical: living in peace.

EXPLANATION: THE OPPOSITE
OF FAT IS LOVE

Remember how the OCD handwashers I talked about in Chapter 8 showed hyperactivity in the area of the brain associated with fear? Well, the place of Thinner Peace seems to have its own little apartments in your gray matter. There's the left prefrontal cortex, where those Tibetan lamas were so well endowed, and which apparently grows larger with every meditating minute. Another brain zone that's switched to "on" by meditation may be the superior posterior parietal lobe. This is what neuroscientists Andrew Newberg and Eugene D'Aquili noticed when they tested accomplished meditators of their own. At the moment the meditating subjects reached a state of deep peace, the superior posterior parietal lobe lit up like a storefront in December.

This bundle of neurons, located toward the back of your head, mediates your sense of what's "you" and what's "not you." Ordinarily, once we're over the age of 2 or 3, we instinctively know that anything inside our skin is us, and the rest of the world isn't. But when the superior posterior parietal lobe is active, that sense of "me, not me" melts away. If you've ever had a moment of feeling utterly connected with the universe, or with another person, this part of your brain was probably contributing to that feeling, if not creating it.

Does this mean that the lover or mystic's sense of oneness with the universe is purely a neural phenomenon? Not necessarily. It could be that the feeling of uniting with The Force is something quite real, which the brain "tunes into" like a radio tuning into a certain station. Since everything we perceive, from an experience of God to an experience of jellybeans, is transmitted by some part of the brain's perceptual apparatus, we have no way of knowing Ultimate Reality. What matters more to me and my ilk is the deep philosophical question: "Will this way of perceiving reality, if developed with focused attention, reliably slenderize my thighs?"

The answer, I have been thrilled to learn, is: Oh, yes. Plus, it feels fabulous, and I mean right now, before you have to lose any weight at all. For those of us who thought we had to starve and discipline ourselves all our lives, this is great news, like realizing you can only get over an excruciating illness by having really great sex. I mean this literally. Newberg and D'Aquili pointed out that the area of the brain they studied may have evolved as a sexual adaptation. In order to mate, individual animals have to allow unusually intimate contact with others, in which body boundaries are temporarily dropped. If this has ever happened to you, you know how powerful it was when the "urge to merge" part of the brain allowed you to feel so psychologically connected to someone else that for a while, your sense of self actually included them: The phrase "you and I are one" was literally subjectively true. In other words, you fell in love.

When I was trying to figure out why some of my clients were losing weight without trying, falling in love turned out to be the common factor. Some tumbled head over heels into romantic relationships and told me that their body fat suddenly seemed to be melting away. Others didn't meet a new person, but as they began living more authentically (something we'll talk about a lot in the coming chapters), they also fell in love with places, activities, professions, works of art, social movements, fields of study, you name it. If they experienced that sense of happy, free-falling, luscious connection, weight loss often seemed to just happen effortlessly—in fact, many people told me that they were actually surprised or mystified by it.

In part, this is because falling in love makes us happy, so we don't do as much "comfort eating." And perhaps our desire to look great naked motivates us to eat less, move more. But I strongly suspect there's something hormonal going on as well. When we're locked in the war between our Dictator and Wild Child selves, our prevailing mental state is anxiety. This causes floods of stress hormones, telling the body to pack in fat supplies, just in case of famine. When we fall in love, our brains start producing hormones associated with mating behavior, the rearing of young, and other noncrisis activities. It's as if the body figures, "Hey, we're in baby-making mode! Things must be pretty good. I can back off the emergency fat storage program." In biological terms, the opposite of getting fat is getting connected, and the antidote to being out of control isn't being in control, but being in love—or, if you want to emphasize the mystical aspect of it, Being in Love, abiding in pure compassion.

Two brain states that are common components of falling in love are appreciation and gratitude. According to medical psychologists, it's neurologically impossible for your brain to create these emotions while simultaneously feeling afraid. Research has shown that focusing on appreciation and gratitude has all kinds of positive health effects, lowering indicators of disease-causing stress and increasing the flow of healthy hormones in our bloodstreams. There are many exercises for triggering this state, none of which I would do merely to reach a boring goal like becoming a better person. However, since they help people lose weight, I do them all. Here are some of my favorite ways to "turn on" appreciation and gratitude, the way you'd turn on a light in a dim space. You can use any or all of them to create your next 4-day win.

EXERCISE: LOVE MEANS NEVER HAVING TO SAY YOU'RE CHUBBY

Create an Appreciation List

To do this exercise, think of someone who's a positive presence in your life. Write down the name of this person

_____

_____

Now, list at least 15 things you appreciate about this individual. You may find that the first couple of items pop easily to mind, after which you'll feel a bit stumped. Keep thinking. Write down *anything* about this person that you appreciate: "She only forgets my name when she's really drunk," or "He's bilaterally symmetrical." Once you push through the slump, you'll find that ideas come easily. According to medical psychologist Dan Baker, you'll also feel your mood improving as your neocortex tells your brain to focus on appreciation. This moves activity from the fearful-reptile zones and triggers the secretion of serotonin, causing feelings of joy.

15 things I appreciate about the person named above:

1. _____

2. _____

3. _____

4. _____

5. _____

6. _____

7. _____

8. _____

9. _____

10. _____

11. _____

12. _____

13. _____

14. _____

15. _____

DO SOME GRATITUDE-GRUBBING

This is a modified form of an exercise recommended by Martin Seligman, former president of the American Psychological Association and a leading practitioner in the field of positive psychology. Once you've listed 15 things in your "appreciation" exercise, write a one-page expression of gratitude to the person you've named. Make an appointment with that person, but don't tell him or her what it's about. Take your one-page paean to the meeting, and read it aloud. To get even more bang for your gratitude buck, do this in front of other people.

TAKE EXTREME MEASURES

If the two previous exercises seem easy, you're ready for the one that shifts your brain activity into happy zones like an earth-mover shoving sand. This exercise is both difficult and simple: Do the "appreciation list" focusing on a person you don't much like. Then do it yet again, finding 15 things to appreciate about someone you actually *dis*like.

You'll find this not only makes you oddly cheerful, but changes your interactions in subtle ways that make your life quite a bit smoother. My experience indicates that people with weight issues often feel judged and attacked, partly because they spend so much time judging and attacking themselves. The resulting defensiveness often triggers other people's paranoia, so that everyone exists in a state of low-level fear and anger. If you're naturally good-natured enough to do these "extreme appreciation" exercises without getting a psychological backlash (see the "I Hate Everybody" option below), they'll transform your relationships as well as your body.

THE "I HATE EVERYBODY" OPTION

If the exercises above make you want to heave, you may have the same kind of jaded, cynical Wild Child I do. Attempting to get all sugary about anyone at all, friend or foe, could trigger a polar bear effect and make you hate everybody. In that case, try this challenge: Name 15 things in your immediate vicinity that are beautiful (to any of your senses). Or, think of 15 experiences in your life for which you are grateful. List these items in the spaces above.

If even this is causing a polar bear–like growling in your mind, be pleased. We have scrounged through your consciousness until we've reached some serious bedrock issues. We have laid bare your thoughts—specifically, the thoughts that are making you fat. Identifying and addressing them can be the most crucial element of transforming your brain into a weight-loss machine.

"Ruthlessly Exploiting Appreciation and Gratitude" 4-Day Win

Ridiculously Easy Daily Goal: *Each day for the next 4 days, I'll write down 15 things I appreciate, or for which I am grateful.*

Small Daily Reward: _____

_____

Slightly Larger 4-Day Reward: _____

_____

	Dates of My Current 4-Day Win	Check Off Completed Days Here
Day 1:	___ / ___ / ___	_____
Day 2:	___ / ___ / ___	_____
Day 3:	___ / ___ / ___	_____
Day 4:	___ / ___ / ___	_____

If you're already on a weight-loss regimen, remember that the 4-day win will enhance it, not conflict with it. If you know what to do, this program will help you do what you know. Feel free to stay on any weight-loss program while you learn 4-day win skills!

CHAPTER 14

HOW NOT TO BE A BIG FAT LIAR

Suppose you and I are sitting in my house, drinking beer and watching the Billiards Channel, when suddenly you notice a huge cobra right by your feet. Aack! You experience an immediate, intense fear response. Aack, aack, aack! Then I burst out laughing, because the cobra is actually a plastic snake I put there to scare you. I poke it to prove it's inanimate. You still feel uneasy, looking at its slick snaky form, but your adrenaline rush probably diminishes. You stop thinking about how to kill the snake and start thinking about how to kill me.

The point is that we don't just react to the world as it is. We react to the world as we think it is—the same coiled black object, identical to the eye, affects us very differently depending on whether we tell ourselves, "That's a snake" or "That's a piece of plastic." We also believe thoughts like "I'm hungry" or "I need pie" even when they aren't true. We react to these inaccurate statements as though they were scientific fact.

As you've gone through the contemplation stage of weight loss, you've learned to align your consciousness with your inner Watcher and perch there, observing your physical and emotional feelings. Just one step remains in your contemplation training—the step that's most profoundly healing and most difficult for a person raised in the rationalist tradition. *You must learn to watch any or all of your thoughts without believing them.* This is a skill that allows you to break away from any psychological conditioning that predisposes you to weight gain. It's a far more useful and effective way to develop a thin person's brain than is traditional psychotherapy.

EXPLANATION: LIES, LIES, LIES!

When I told one client that a lot of her beliefs about her own limitations were untrue, she said, "Oh, so now I'm a big fat liar?" No, of course she wasn't. Neither are you. You're a very honest person, except for that unfortunate college incident involving the dean's boxer-briefs and 14 ounces of superglue. But we buy into a lot of cultural lies told by folks who honestly believe them, and our unwitting acceptance of these fibs can keep us from thinking thin.

I'm a big fan of psychotherapy, which helped me see through a huge number of lies I'd told myself for years—lies like "Anger is always wrong" or "Righteous people don't enjoy sex" or "There is a rogue Secret Service agent dressed as a French maid who follows me everywhere, waiting for a chance to stun me with a tranquilizer dart and sell my organs to the Soviet Union." (My therapist explained to me that the Soviet Union no longer exists. Silly me!)

As I've worked with overweight people and compulsive eaters, I've noticed that most of them hold certain patterns of inaccurate beliefs, many of which they've absorbed, by capillary action, from the very psychotherapeutic tradition I revere. Believing these lies is totally understandable in our culture, but ultimately they are disempowering. Unless you articulate and examine them, you may one day find yourself salting, peppering, and consuming the leather interior of your new luxury convertible. And that would be a shame.

THE EASY WAY THAT ISN'T EASY

There's an old joke about a wealthy woman who gets out of her limo at the Ritz Carlton and asks for two bellmen, one to carry her luggage, the other to haul her 10-year-old son. The bellman picks up the child, whose legs are pitifully withered, and says to the woman, "Ma'am, it's such a pity your son can't walk." To which the woman replies, "Well, of course he can walk! But, thank God, he'll never have to!"

The lie that motivated this woman was that her boy's life would be easier if everything was done *for* him. This is what I call the EASY myth. EASY stands for "External Authority System: You." The myth is that if an external authority system cares for us—in other words, if someone not "me" but "you" is running my life—everything will be great. This belief makes us look for weight loss as something we can get from something or someone else: a diet book, a doctor, a coach, a dietitian, a lover, an exercise program. If that external source of authority works correctly, we'll lose weight and be happy.

This logic is excellent except that it never, ever works. The reality is that if external systems govern us, we wither. We are not empowered but disempowered by anything that does for us what we can do for ourselves. It was easier for Christopher Reeve's body to have all its breathing done for it after a terrible accident left him a quadriplegic. His lungs didn't have to work—the machines did it all. Was his life easier? In a strict sense of energy exerted, the answer is yes, but of course that's absurd. *There are things we are meant to do ourselves, and when these things are done for us, the result is suffering. Weight loss is one of these things.*

I often have overweight clients who are angry that their parents didn't teach them to eat better, that their mothers gave them food when they were sad, that their personal trainer charged too much and therefore "forced" them to give up exercise, or that the antichocolate diet book they believed in so deeply did not physically prevent them from snuffling truffles. It's terrible to trust a system and find that it doesn't work, and I empathize with these people's disappointment. But the reality is that external authority systems (EASY weight-loss strategies) always ultimately fail. At best, they give you a temporary sense of exultant security followed by a sickening disillusionment, like marrying a charming sociopath.

In order to be a thin person, you have to exchange your belief in the EASY weight-loss myth with what I call the CALM reality. Where EASY stands for "External Authority System: You," CALM stands for "Compassionate, Authoritative Learning: Me." You'll lose weight when you realize that kindly attending to your own internal needs and wants, both physical and emotional, is the only way to stay lean and healthy. *You are the ultimate authority on you. No one else can ever claim that authority, and you cannot give it away, even if you want to.*

When I talk about picking up authority for one's own life, a lightbulb goes on for many of my overweight clients. Just articulating unconscious beliefs helps them see where they've given up their authority over their own bodies. Below, I've listed the most powerful and common EASY fibs, along with CALM insights that actually will help you stay thin forever. There are 12 EASY beliefs I call the "dirty dozen." The CALM insights I've cited to challenge these fibs aren't gospel truth. Don't simply swallow them whole. Instead, consider each one and see what part of it, if any, rings true for you. *This process—seeing what rings true, dismissing everything else—is what centers and grounds you in your own authority. It's an essential skill for being skinny and healthy.* Weighing the evidence is the equivalent of walking or breathing on your own: It may be easier to have it done for you, but thank God, you get to do it on your own.

EASY Versus CALM: Dodging the Dirty Dozen and Staying Grounded in Reality

EASY Myth #1: The power to make me thin and keep me thin is hidden in some exogenous authority source: a book, a trainer, a doctor, a parent, a coach, a program, a product.

CALM Insight #1: When I am relaxed and feeling comfortable in my skin, I can choose healthy behaviors without triggering famine reactions. I may not yet understand how to stay relaxed, but certainly no one else can do it for me.

EASY Myth #2: To lose weight, I must absolutely comply with my external authority source (diet, trainer, program) the way a child complies with a parent. It is the external authority's job to initiate activity, notice when I need more support of any kind and deliver the right support in the right way, and sustain my discipline. In other words, my job is to be the perfect child. My authority source's job is to be the perfect parent.

CALM Insight #2: When I was very young, complying with authority really was my only way of staying safe and figuring out how the world works. But now that I'm capable of analyzing reality on my own, playing a child role is frustrating and makes me feel powerless. Something in me is telling me that I get to be the grown-up in my life and that if I *totally* comply with any external system, I'll end up giving away my autonomy, individuality, and self-respect. My instincts tell me when to question. If I listen to them, I won't feel or act like a trapped and angry child.

EASY Myth #3: A perfect weight-loss authority source will eliminate the possibility of my breaking the rules.

CALM Insight #3: The only thing that creates total compliance is total dependency. Prisoners and people with total paralysis or extreme illness are the only adults who can't choose to disobey. Far from creating happiness, the loss of autonomous choice is horrible. It's the single variable most related to depression and despair. I'm grateful that I have the choice to break the rules of my fitness program, because the alternative is loss of all personal power.

EASY Myth #4: The way to free myself from the negative influence of flawed authority sources is to discuss them for a very long time with better people. Then, these new people will be the perfect authority sources, and they can take over the job of managing any feelings and actions that cause weight gain.

CALM Insight #4: Though it really helps to talk through beliefs that came from powerful people in my life and though healthier people really can help me see things differently, once I've identified and articulated the problems, rehashing them over and over doesn't change much. What changes me is *questioning beliefs that feel wrong and seeking within myself a belief that feels more true.* Once I have learned to question a flawed set of rules, the next step is to break those rules and see if that works better for me. Loved ones and counselors can support me, but changing my life requires behaving differently, not just discussing the reasons for dysfunctional behavior.

EASY Myth #5: When I finally locate the perfect human to be my authority source, I'll feel so cared for that all anger, fear, and sadness will disappear from my emotional landscape. Then I won't eat for comfort.

CALM Insight #5: The most basic structure in the human noggin, the so-called "reptilian brain," is designed to be hypersensitive to lack and attack. No matter how loving and powerful your human authority source, the ups and downs of your life will continue. (I know many people who meet the perfect lover and then immediately begin obsessing about losing that person.) Fortunately, there are humans who have learned to gently school their own brains so that they, themselves, can step out of fear, anger, and sadness and see it from the perspective of complete compassion. These methods, not perfect parental figures, are my only ticket to lasting slenderness.

EASY Myth #6: Just as someone external to me must be my source for emotional nourishment, I must be the perfect source of emotional nourishment for others. I owe it to those I love to make life EASY for them.

CALM Insight #6: Thinking I should make others feel good or be healthy is like the rich woman thinking she can save her son from distress by hiring people to carry him around. Each being is born with the burden and privilege of becoming his or her own ultimate source of authority. I can put down the burden of unhealthy caretaking.

EASY Myth #7: Once the perfect EASY system is in place, with others supplying my needs and determining my behavior while I supply and manage my loved ones' lives, there will be no possibility of going back. Everything will work perfectly from then on.

CALM Insight #7: Learning never ends, and no condition is permanent. But life without change or challenge would be like life in a rubber room. The way to cope with life's constant change and uncertain progress is to relish fresh experiences, not avoid them.

EXERCISE: YOUR FOOD-MOOD-BROOD JOURNAL

Practically every body of research on slenderizing reminds us that keeping a food journal is a powerful tool for weight loss. Most researchers seem to assume that this is because being aware of our food intake—how many calories? how many carbs?—makes us more compliant with external authority. I think a more powerful reason is that observation activates the Watcher in our brains and helps us question our erroneous assumptions. On the following page, you'll find a form you can copy and use to create an especially fabulous and detailed sort of eating journal. I call it your "Food-Mood-Brood" record because it has spaces for notes on food and for the feelings and thoughts you had while you were eating.

Your Food-Mood-Brood Contemplation Journal

To achieve maximum contemplation power, make several copies of this page, put them in a binder, and use them to keep a careful record of what you eat, feel, and think.

TIME OF DAY	WHAT I ATE	HUNGER LEVEL (-10 TO +10)	WHAT I WAS FEELING PHYSICALLY	WHAT I WAS FEELING EMOTIONALLY	THOUGHT I WAS THINKING	REASON THAT THOUGHT MAY NOT BE TRUE

As you look over the thoughts and emotions that fueled your eating, see if any of them reflect the "dirty dozen" assumptions of the EASY mythology. Please remember that these thought patterns come from our culture, and you needn't ever judge or blame yourself for having them. But if you do notice the dirty dozen creeping into your thoughts about eating and weight, read over the CALM insights, and see if anything in them resonates with your sense of truth. If not, come up with some other alternative that does feel true for you. *Because you are the authority figure in your life. Not this book, not your spouse, not your parents, not Drs. Atkins, Pritikin, or Doolittle. You.* If you've been weakened by some of the lies that make weight loss seem impossible, it's time to get up and flex your mental powers. The food-mood-brood journal 4-day win is the place to do it. Learning to disentangle your eating from cultural myths is a forefield skill, so you may want to do this 4-day win often.

"Food-Mood-Brood Journal"
4-Day Win

Ridiculously Easy Daily Goal: *Each day for the next 4 days, I'll keep my food-mood-brood journal to see what thoughts and emotions are linked to my overeating. I'll reread any of the EASY myths that I may have internalized and see what CALM insights feel right to me.* _____

Small Daily Reward: _____

_____

Slightly Larger 4-Day Reward: _____

_____

	Dates of My Current 4-Day Win	Check Off Completed Days Here
Day 1:	___ / ___ / ___	_____
Day 2:	___ / ___ / ___	_____
Day 3:	___ / ___ / ___	_____
Day 4:	___ / ___ / ___	_____

If you're already on a weight-loss regimen, remember that the 4-day win will enhance it, not conflict with it. If you know what to do, this program will help you do what you know. Feel free to stay on any weight-loss program while you learn 4-day win skills!

CHAPTER 15

NOT ALWAYS SO: FROM FATHEAD TO OPEN MIND

I first noticed my emotional-eating triggers at the movies. I'd get to the theater, sit down, and munch some popcorn, maybe a couple of Junior Mints for dessert. I'd be sick of grease, salt, and sugar by the time the movie started. Then I'd get caught up in the story of eight guys trying to blow up an asteroid, or two lovers making out on a ship, or a bunch of penguins trying to keep their eggs from freezing. One day I noticed that whenever something in the movie made me even slightly upset, I'd grab for my popcorn bag as if it were the emergency oxygen mask on a depressurizing passenger jet.

Thought: That asteroid is getting mighty close to the earth. Response: Eat.

Thought: The *Titanic* just hit the iceberg! Response: Eat!

Thought: *Oh, my God, the egg broke!* Response: *Eat! Eat! Eat!*

Of course this isn't logical. It's bio-logical. Engrossed in a movie, I have the same fight-or-flight reaction that helped trigger food hoarding and fat accumulation when my cave-ancestors were under direct physical threat. Our bodies don't know from movies. Horrified by the death of Bambi's mother or the latest chainsaw massacre, they get right to work flooding us with stress hormones and preparing us to survive the imminent food shortage, all in reaction to projected images flickering on a screen.

The ultimate takeaway from becoming a contemplative—learning to see your own mind and body so clearly that you're not dragged into involuntary responses like overeating—is this startling realization: *All thoughts are projected images flickering on a screen.* Our lives are stories we write, direct, record, edit, and view within the confines of our internal perceptual apparatus. It's inevitable and normal to see our lives as narratives of our own creation, but it becomes a problem when we mistake the stories in our minds for The Truth. When those stories get upsetting, those of us with weight issues can put away enough Junior Mints to comprise a very large Senior Mint.

In the last chapter, I asked you to contemplate the degree to which you've believed and internalized cultural myths about authority, particularly when it comes to weight loss. I encouraged you to challenge those lies. Now I want you to go spelunking a little more deeply into your psyche to see if you've been telling yourself other kinds of lies—and whether those affect your emotions and the way you eat.

You've heard the term "emotional eating," because most diet experts now know that this is a major factor that keeps people fat. What you may not have heard is that emotion isn't the fundamental problem. Many of my clients spend years in therapy talking about their emotions, thinking that eventually, this will help them eliminate emotional eating. It rarely does. Why not? Because the fundamental problem is your mind, not your emotions. Emotions are virtually always responses to thoughts. That's great news, because *while it's impossible to control an emotion once a thought has triggered it, we can change our thoughts deliberately. We do this not by contradicting them, but by questioning them.*

EXPLANATION: FATTENING FEARS

An enormous amount of research points to the connection between believing our own negative thoughts and a host of dysfunctional consequences, from depression to illness to addiction. All of these factors affect our relationship with food. They also change the hormonal balance that mediates things like hunger and fat accumulation. After years of working with overweight clients, I've observed that *the psychological variable most linked to obesity isn't weakness, laziness, lack of commitment, or inadequate motivation. It's an unwillingness to question thoughts that cause anxiety.*

Some psychologists recommend that dieters repeat affirmations, like "My diet of celery and Bingo cards is satisfying and delicious!" But because such thoughts are inauthentic and externally imposed—and because the body hates to lie—they often create horrific polar-bear reactions. You might as well have Hostess Twinkies injected directly into your buttocks. No, becoming naturally thin requires not attaching to new thoughts but opening our minds.

It's been said that the entire philosophical foundation of Zen is contained in three small words: "Not always so." If you want to stop emotional eating (which means you'll eat only out of physical hunger, which means you'll eventually be the right weight for your body) you must become willing to apply those three words to your own beliefs.

THE LIES WE LIVE BY

Does questioning your thoughts sound easy? It is, in a strictly procedural sense, but when it comes to the way our egos work, it's actually a challenge. Admitting that our thoughts may be in error demands humility—not the self-hatred many plump people possess in industrial quantities, but the genuine willingness to admit that we're human and that therefore we make mistakes. Lao Tzu wrote, "All streams flow to the sea because it is lower than they are. Humility gives it its power." Empowering ourselves to lose weight requires relinquishing the conviction that the stories we tell ourselves are The Truth and seeing them instead as arbitrary mental constructions.

Take Dave, the diabetic lawyer who shoveled in all those suicidal doughnuts at a wedding banquet. A few days after the binge, once we got him calmed down and identified with his Watcher self, Dave was able to observe in memory the very moment he headed into his binge-trance. It was the moment when he'd said to himself, "I have to go to Amelia's wedding now."

Obviously, this was a big, huge, scary lie.

Huh? Most people disagree with me when I say things like this. They think that the statement "I have to go to Amelia's wedding now" is reasonable, true, and certainly not terrifying. I disagree.

First of all, it's true that Dave was *expected* to go to the wedding—Amelia was his niece, so a lot of people would have noticed if he hadn't shown up. But he didn't literally *have to*. He could have spent the whole day fishing, or planting rutabaga, or hiding under a bridge. Would this have been socially awkward? No question. But was it physically possible? Yes, indeed. Dave was perfectly capable of skipping the wedding. When I point out this kind of thing to a client who's significantly overweight, I expect a bloody battle, and

I'm rarely disappointed. The more a client struggles with weight, the more passionately he or she will defend statements like, "I have to go to the wedding," "I can't skip work," "I've got to pay the rent," "I have to be there for my children," "I have to lose weight," etc., etc. All lies.

You may be feeling indignant right now, thinking these statements are often undeniably true. That's because you not only believe them, but *fear disbelieving* them. We get furious when someone questions our fear-based assumptions because such thoughts are based on our most powerfully reinforced social training, and when we flout social norms we risk ostracism, shame, perhaps even isolation. We're afraid disaster will ensue if we stopped believing these little lies, and as long as we believe them, we're afraid to act as though they may not be true. "Of course I have to lose weight!" my chubby clients shout, almost panicky. "Everybody thinks so! My doctor says so! I'll die of heart disease if I don't!"

Maybe. But the statement "I have to lose weight" is still a lie.

I'm not questioning that losing weight can be healthy, nor the assertion that everybody thinks you're fat. I'm just saying that in a literal sense, the statement "I have to lose weight" is untrue because it's possible for you *not* to lose weight. It's not true that you're physically incapable of skipping work, refusing to pay rent, and so on. You choose to do these things to avoid negative consequences. Strange as it may seem, the way you word this, in your own mind, has a huge impact on your ability to drop excess weight and stay lean.

If you think this is mere hairsplitting, you haven't read much about linguistic epistemology—the study of the way language helps create the way we know our reality. This research shows that to your psyche and your body, messages like "I can't" and "I have to" are worlds apart from phrases like "I'm going to" or "I choose to." Untruths that roll blithely off our tongues lodge in our tissues like a witch's spell. A life lived according to inaccurate beliefs, no matter how innocent, is a life ruled by fear. And to the extent that our lives are ruled by fear, we have an insanely difficult time staying thin.

For example, when Dave thought the innocent little sentence, "I have to go to Amelia's wedding," his body reacted as though this were literally true—as though he had no options and no escape. This drove his Wild Child into a frenzy of fear and rage, which is any creature's response to being trapped and helpless. The panic and rage he felt because he believed himself to be helpless fueled Dave's binge. He would have experienced the whole evening differently if he'd thought, "I guess I'll go to this wedding, since I want to be there for my niece, but I could do other things with that time if I chose." Even days later, when Dave dropped the first belief and stated the second, he felt a wave of relief, and his compulsivity about eating dropped a level. The difference between "I have to," and "I guess I will" was the difference between normal eating and a bingeing warp spasm.

You can learn to see past the lies that blind by doing the following exercises.

EXERCISE: NOT ALWAYS SO

1. Link Behavior with the Lies That Drive It

Sit down with a notebook and a writing implement. Draw a vertical line down the middle of the paper. Then relax, access your Watcher, and observe your physical/emotional state until you see a relaxation response. Return in memory to a time you overate. Sit with the memory until you can recall the thoughts you were thinking as you ate. If you pay close attention, you'll see that there is always a thought underlying the decision to eat, though it may not have been articulated. Articulate it now. The thought that made you eat for escape could be almost anything, such as, "I've got to pay the bills," "I need to walk the dogs," or "I really should give Bernice my kidney." Whatever it is, identify it and write it down on the left-hand side of the page.

2: Question Your Thoughts

Once you've committed the thought to paper, repeat it in your mind a few times and notice that thinking it creates anxiety. Now, on the right-hand side of the page, write down at least one reason the original thought may not be true. Don't replace it with a contradictory thought, insisting "That's wrong! This is right!" Just think of some possible way the thought *might* not be *absolutely* true. Do it as a logic problem. Say to yourself, "The sentence, 'I've got to pay the bills' is overstating the case. 'I choose to pay the bills' is closer to the truth." Instead of "I need to walk the dogs" you might say, "I'm going to walk the dogs, because they love taking walks, and I love them." Point out to yourself, "I'm under a lot of pressure to give Bernice a kidney, but the choice is mine."

EXAMPLE OF THOUGHT-QUESTIONING EXERCISE

What I ate: Some cake. Actually, a cake.

THOUGHT THAT FUELED MY OVEREATING	WHY THIS THOUGHT MAY NOT ALWAYS BE SO
My son Spike got fired from his job at the body-piercing den. He's going to end up moving back home. and I'll have to support him forever. Him and his piercings.	It's possible Spike wasn't fired. He may have quit, then lied about it. Also, I can decide not to let him move back home. It would be emotionally hard, but it's possible.

Remember: *The idea here is not to change your behavior, only to open your mind.* This is one of the 4-day wins that I really want you to try, since it will help you feel a subtle sense of relaxation and empowerment that will form the new core of your worldview. Learning to challenge the thoughts in your head is a forefield skill, one you may want to use quite often, even daily, whenever you catch yourself feeling stuck and disempowered because you think something must be true. Using this new way of thinking, you can build an entire way of life that will make controlling your weight easier than it has ever been.

"Not Always So" 4-Day Win

Ridiculously Easy Daily Goal: *Each day for the next 4 days, I'll write down things I've eaten when not hungry. I'll sit with the memory until I can identify the thought that triggered the eating. Then I'll think of at least one reason, no matter how far-fetched, that my triggering thought may not always be so.*

Small Daily Reward: _____

_____

Slightly Larger 4-Day Reward: _____

_____

	Dates of My Current 4-Day Win	**Check Off Completed Days Here**
Day 1:	___/___/___	_____
Day 2:	___/___/___	_____
Day 3:	___/___/___	_____
Day 4:	___/___/___	_____

If you're already on a weight-loss regimen, remember that the 4-day win will enhance it, not conflict with it. If you know what to do, this program will help you do what you know. Feel free to stay on any weight-loss program while you learn 4-day win skills!

CHAPTER 16

BEWARE THE PERMANENTLY HELPLESS DALMATIAN REPTILE

The more you do the "contemplation" exercises you've been learning, the sooner you'll heal the psychological wounds wrought by dieting, and thus increase your ability to get thin and stay that way. Of course, you won't be able to sustain a state of serenity every second—no one can, not even contemplatives who make serenity their full-time job. You'll slip into old thought patterns and behaviors, succumbing to stress, falling prey to mildly delusional fears, and overeating, again and again. That's absolutely fine, as long as you persistently return to the identity of the Watcher, question your own beliefs, and calm your body.

Remember those Tibetan monks, whose brains were literally denser in areas related to happiness? By returning, returning, and returning again to a place of peace, they built their neurological capacity for joy and calm. It's similar to the way a weightlifter builds muscle by repeatedly lifting the same weight—the point isn't to get the weight to stay up in the air, but the act of lifting itself. So don't worry that you'll have to pull yourself out of old thought-ruts many times: the more you do it, the more you'll feel yourself undergoing metamorphosis, leaving caterpillar life behind, sensing that you'll soon have wings.

The last two chapters showed you how your creature-brain reacts to the lies it hears by overeating; this chapter describes how your verbal mind compiles all those little lies into some typical grander storylines as it constructs your experience of life. As you observe the thoughts that drive overeating, you'll notice that they tend to add up to habitual storylines, narrative plots by which you both understand and create your experience of life. Research shows that folks who tend toward chubbiness share a few typical mental storylines, and therefore, it's helpful to be prepared to recognize them when you see them. The more quickly you spot them, the faster you can escape from the stress and angst that will make your life a frustrating festival of fat.

ADIPOSE ASSUMPTIONS

In *The Sixth Sense,* director M. Night Shyamalan managed to pull off a dramatic surprise ending by capitalizing on moviegoers' assumptions that we know a lot of things we actually don't. I won't ruin the movie for readers who haven't seen it, but I can say that Shyamalan shows little bits of action in the characters' lives and lets us "fill in" the rest of the story with unconscious assumptions. Only in the last few minutes does the script reveal that these assumptions are way off the mark.

Life is a lot like that.

We can't possibly know everything about reality—every tiny fact about every situation, every little event that's occurring in every place we go. So our brains collect the information they think is most important, and "fill in" the rest with imagination and supposition. People with weight issues tend to fill in knowledge gaps with similar assumptions. The worst culprits are:

1. The illusion of fixed conditions
2. Learned helplessness
3. Dichotomous thinking
4. The lack/attack syndrome

These are very, very fattening ways of thinking. Watch out for them. If you can cut these storylines out of your brain's thought menu (by questioning them and seeing their inaccuracy) you'll be much healthier physically—and psychologically.

1. The Illusion of Fixed Conditions

Nothing is permanent. This is one of Buddhism's "noble truths," and we're all aware of it. Yet we—especially those of us with weight issues—

speak as if things are fixed in time. Dieters think in terms of "being" fat, "being" on a diet, and then "being" thin. It's more accurate to think of the body as ever-changing: we get bigger or smaller every moment of every day, and losing weight is about moving the whole statistical process toward eating less and moving more.

The most fascinating study on this topic is one in which subjects lost an average of 11 pounds after making just one behavioral change: they stopped using any form of the verb "to be." Try this yourself: describe your weight history (your recollections of your struggle to get or stay thin) without using words like "is," "are," "am," "was," "has been," "will be," "hasn't been," "won't be," "were," "weren't," "isn't," "aren't," etc.

Description of my weight history without any form of the verb "to be":

_____

_____

_____

Not easy, is it? To do this, you have to start using phrases like, "My body carries a lot of fat," or "I hope one day I can look in the mirror and see one lean Marine. Also myself." This wording removes our identification with a fixed condition and allows us to perceive the freedom to change. The statement "I am fat," equates "fat" with being, with existence. If "I am fat," then not having fat means not existing (bad thing). If my body simply "carries" a lot of extra tissue, losing it means putting down a burden (good thing).

This study dovetails with research on "explanatory style," in which scientists noted that the way people explain the events of their lives has a powerful effect on various physical indicators of health. People whose thought patterns explain negative events as permanent, personal, and pervasive ("I'll always be fat because it's just my rotten luck") have relatively bad health and trouble achieving goals. Since explaining events this way not only increases weight-related pathologies but also predicts failure in everything from earning money to running for office, the technical term for people who talk this way should probably be "big fat losers." On the other hand, people who see negative events as being transitory ("I'm getting a little hefty since I started this job. Time to take off some weight.") were more able to reach their goals, had much better physical health, and lived longer.

I've seen first-hand how releasing the assumption of fixed conditions helps my clients feel better about themselves, lose weight more quickly, and keep it off more easily. As for verb usage being the single factor necessary to lose weight . . . well, this study hasn't been replicated enough to make me a true believer, but let's just say I carry a lot of optimism about it.

2. Learned Helplessness

The informal guru of positive psychology, Martin Seligman, rose to fame on the backs of helpless dogs. Or, to be more accurate, dogs who thought they were helpless, even though they actually weren't.

Seligman spent years sticking canines in various cages, harnesses, and hammocks, then giving them electric shocks. Some of the dogs could stop or avoid the shocks by jumping over a low divider or pressing a lever. Others had no control; they got shocked no matter what they did. When the second group of dogs was moved over to new situations where they could avoid the shocks, they didn't do anything. One little hop over the divider, and they would have been safe, but because they'd learned to expect that nothing they did would help, they just sat there and suffered. The other dogs, who hadn't learned to feel helpless, immediately and successfully avoided the shocks. These dogs showed no noticeable behavior changes while Seligman's accounts of these experiments said that the dogs with learned helplessness "showed signs of clinical depression." I assume this entailed moping, shedding, and singing "Don't Cry Out Loud" while eating pint after pint of rum raisin ice cream. But I may just be projecting.

In my opinion, there's no experience worse than dieting for giving humans a sense of learned helplessness. You starve yourself for months on end, then lose control and binge like crazy while your lowered metabolism makes you inflate like a parade balloon, and everyone starts thinking you're ugly and lazy. Just writing about it makes me lose hair. That's why it's so important for overweight people to learn the real mechanics of weight loss. You really were helpless to lose weight when your only method was voluntary self-starvation. But you're not anymore. If you change your approach, you really can reshape your body. Believing that you can find a way to fix your life—size being just one component—is key to both successful weight loss and overall happiness.

3. Dichotomous Thinking

My dear friend Annette has lived on the diet roller coaster for as long as I've known her. The way she loses weight is simple: she goes off food. For months. After entire seasons adhering to some medically supervised liquid diet, she starts showing subtle signs of malnutrition, such as passing out and falling over. This causes her to consider the wacky idea that she might actually benefit from eating something. So she'll buy several of her favorite bakery-fresh cookies, and eat them all at once.

The other day I said to Annette, who had consumed nothing but green tea for a week, "What would you think about eating until your body felt satisfied, and then stopping?"

"What are you?" she said, appalled, "Some kind of terrorist?"

I'm not sure why the idea of gray areas is so upsetting to someone who repeatedly looks starvation in the face with nary a flinch. What I do know is that Annette's thought style, known to psychologists as "dichotomous thinking," is highly correlated with unwanted weight. My friends at the Jenny Craig weight-loss company, spend a lot of time trying to figure out how to help customers stop thinking solely in black and white terms. But most dieters are bafflingly resistant.

I think this is because the fight-or-flight part of the brain is predisposed to thinking in dual opposites. Western philosophies, including the Big Three monotheistic religions (Christianity, Judaism, and Islam) not to mention the more modern faith of rationalism, reinforce this black-and-white, right-or-wrong world view. My favorite Asian philosopher, Lao Tzu, pointed out the inherent danger in this tendency more than 2,500 years ago when he observed:

> Whether you go up the ladder or down it,
> your position is shaky . . .
> See the world as yourself.
> Have faith in the way things are.

In dieter's terms, whether the scale's going up or down, dichotomous thinking makes it inevitable you'll end up pudgy. I know all too well the manic intensity of going on a rigid eating program and hanging onto it like a lifeline, afraid that one illicit potato chip would catapult me off the narrow ladder of success. I also know the horrifying sense of losing my grip on that ladder, falling into compulsive overeating and weight gain, wondering how the hell I lost the discipline I'd thought would solve the problem forever. If you resist something, you end up strengthening it.

Lao Tzu's solution ("See the world as yourself. Have faith in the way things are.") may seem odd, vague, or ineffectual, but it squares with everything we've been learning about the human brain. I think he was referring to the mindset of stepping off the repression/overindulgence ladder, returning to the balanced compassion of the Watcher, achieving the "in love" sensation that dissolves the separation between self and everything. Forget metaphysics: When we let go of the damaging idea that the world can be only this way or that, our brains and hormones can go into a mode where we feel bliss, gain confidence, and find it much easier to lose weight.

4. The Lack-Attack Syndrome

Your reptilian brain holds two fear-based assumptions in its scaly grip. The first assumption says, "There won't be enough for me." Not enough food, love, shelter, not enough anything. The second one frets, "Something bad is about to happen." Someone's out to get me, I'm about to be struck by lightning, a sociopath disguised as my grandmother is planning to add my collarbones to her collection.

You inherited lack-and-attack fears because they're so useful to a lizard on the open veld. Research has shown that fearful people often experience this sense of dread without any actual cause, then search their environments for reasons to justify that fear. Television news capitalizes on our obsession with lack-and-attack fears and also gives us plenty of justification for persistent anxiety. I have clients who tell me they can't possibly stop being actively afraid of anthrax attacks or social injustice, given what they see on the news. But the days they really get hysterical are those when they don't even see the news, and their fearful imaginations run wilder than ever.

Paradoxically, lack-and-attack fears often lead us to put ourselves in danger in the interest of staying safe. Take, for example, Martha Stewart. I'd bet it was lack-and-attack anxiety that motivated her to cheat and then lie about what was (for her) a ridiculously small sum of money. This eventually landed her in prison—all because her knee-jerk reaction, like most people's, was to scurry around defending her fortune and reputation. Is it a coincidence that this incredibly disciplined, smart, perfectionistic, image-conscious woman had also put on weight in the years prior to her prison stay? I think not.

Lack-and-attack thinking often shows up as constant worry, anxiety, complaining, hostility, and sometimes outright panic. It ruins your quality of life, motivates overeating, raises your stress hormones to dangerous levels. The bad news is that we can't eliminate our "Inner Lizard" lack-and-attack center; it's hard-wired right into the base of our brains. The good news is that we can notice it and soothe it.

If you notice yourself lapsing into lack-and-attack mode, use the exercise from the last chapter: Write down your scary thoughts and question them. Are they literally true? Then go to your treasure chest for a memory that sparks gratitude or appreciation. This, not panic or anxiety, will make your world a safer place. Once you've taken all the action you can to prevent global warming or terrorism or the demise of your entire family in a freak accident at the Macy's Thanksgiving Day Parade, worrying about these things does nothing but make you fat and miserable.

EXERCISE: WARDING OFF THE DALMATIAN REPTILE

You can avoid the fallout from these four storylines by simply noticing they're there, calming yourself, going to your inner Watcher, and turning on your love responses in place of fattening thoughts. As a kind of shorthand, remember the phrase "Beware the Permanently Helpless Dalmatian Reptile." The key words are "permanent" (the illusion of fixed states) "helpless" (learned helplessness) "dalmatian" (black and white) and "reptile" (your reptilian brain's lack-and-attack fears).

To see where your patterns most often emerge, complete the sentences in the box on page 126 with the first words that come to mind. Don't overthink this by putting in answers you think are "right" in the context of this book. Just put down your knee-jerk reaction, because that's how we'll figure out where your most troublesome thought patterns tend to focus.

Most likely, all the sentences as you just completed them are untrue. If you kindly and patiently examine each one, you'll find that you're used to exaggerating the permanency of situations or conditions, your own helplessness, the absoluteness of moral judgments, and the threats you face in your everyday life. That just means you're human. Some of us focus more on our fears, others on black-and-white dichotomies, still others on being "helplessly

PERMANENTLY HELPLESS DALMATIAN REPTILE DETECTION

1. I need to worry about _____

2. I get stuck because _____

3. I have to _____

4. I've never had enough _____

5. It would be a disaster if I _____

6. I can't ever let myself _____

7. I can't tolerate people who _____

8. It's always wrong to _____

9. I mustn't _____

10. I shouldn't ever _____

11. I always _____

12. I am _____

stuck" in circumstances that are actually transitory or avoidable.

Use the contemplative skill of questioning to deal with your own set of issues. Think of a reason each sentence you completed above might not always be absolutely true. Like the 4-day wins for the Food-Mood-Brood Journal and Questioning Whether It's Always So, the Permanently Helpless Dalmatian Reptile 4-day win will help you develop a forefield skill you'll use often. Use these skills to remain in the position of the questioner, the Watcher, as you move on to the capstone contemplation exercise in the next chapter.

"Permanently Helpless Dalmatian Reptile" 4-Day Win

Ridiculously Easy Daily Goal: _Each day for the next 4 days, I'll search my own thoughts for Permanently Helpless Dalmatian Reptile storylines, question these thoughts, and re-focus on gratitude or appreciation._ _____

Small Daily Reward: _____

_____

Slightly Larger 4-Day Reward: _____

_____

	Dates of My Current 4-Day Win	**Check Off Completed Days Here**
Day 1:	____ / ____ / ____	_____
Day 2:	____ / ____ / ____	_____
Day 3:	____ / ____ / ____	_____
Day 4:	____ / ____ / ____	_____

If you're already on a weight-loss regimen, remember that the 4-day win will enhance it, not conflict with it. If you know what to do, this program will help you do what you know. Feel free to stay on any weight-loss program while you learn 4-day win skills!

CHAPTER 17

RESEARCHING YOUR LIFE

YOUR WEIGHT LIFELINE

If you've actually been doing the exercises and 4-day wins that suit your psyche up to this point, you've learned to trigger and sustain the brain and body changes that will turn you into a naturally thin person. Those exercises are powerful weight-loss tools, but they don't require any external activity; they all happen in your head. As you're becoming contemplative, learning to watch your own life, you've probably also begun to notice that certain external conditions—people, places, situations—are more likely to make you overeat, while others may actually make it easier to stop overeating.

This is why fitness gurus are always telling us that weight is about lifestyle, not just diet. By lifestyle, I mean not just a new fitness program but your entire daily routine—the amount and type of work you do, the people with whom you hang out, the weather in the place where you live. I've often watched clients' weight rise or drop when they alter lifestyle components (quitting a job, making a new friend) that have no direct connection to either food or exercise. It's like creating a setting for a jewel. Your perfect body is the jewel, the setting is your life. Until the setting is ready to hold the jewel, it won't stay where you want it.

In this last contemplation exercise, we're going to step up the intensity and specificity of your research on your own lifestyle. Then you'll have all the information you need to begin Stage 3 of the transtheoretical model of change, preparation, wherein you make external changes to create and sustain permanent healthy skinniness. Your actual weight-loss efforts—

eating less, moving more—will rely on the changes you make to prepare for them.

EXPLANATION: THE HISTORY OF YOU

Sue is about as active a 55-year-old as you're likely to find. She works at a summer camp for middle school students, where she spends all day navigating ropes courses, climbing rocks, gathering firewood, and restraining herself from smacking obnoxious adolescents. She's always been thin, with maybe just the slightest bit of cellulite on her hindquarters. That is, until last year.

"I don't know why I can't take off this weight," she says of the 30 extra pounds she's added in the past few months. "I think I'm eating the same. I'm still active."

At my suggestion, Sue dutifully checks with her doctors, who test her reproductive hormones, her thyroid, and every other medical factor they can think of. When all the tests come back normal, I begin to suspect that Sue's problems are situational rather than physiological. I assign her some personal research by doing something I call a "weight history lifeline." Using a grid like the one you'll find in the following pages, she estimated how chubby (or not) she was throughout her life.

This process made it clear that Sue gained weight whenever she was involved with a man in trouble. Two former boyfriends, one husband, and Sue's adult son had all experienced rough times related to health, alcohol, or debt. In each case, Sue had taken on extra work to help them get by and had taken care of them psychologically while they groused about their illness, their trouble with sobriety, their financial frustration.

Interestingly, the fat Sue gained during these times clung to her belly, which was unusual for her. She was typically a pear, not an apple, with extra pounds settling in her rear and thighs. Belly fat is often a signal that the body is creating a lot of stress hormones. The combination of man trouble and tummy fat suggested that Sue's excess weight was related to the way she dealt with male loved ones. Before the classic eat-less-move-more combination would work well, Sue had to address her central unconscious lie: "I have to keep my men out of trouble."

When Sue finally began to question this belief, it occurred to her that many of these menfolk had actually asked her to butt out and let them live their own lives. She hadn't done so because the deep-seated unconscious lie had overwritten their requests. Now that she recognized it, she could change it. After weeks of observing her own behavior regarding money, men, and food, Sue came to the conclusion that she'd feel better if she designated a certain portion of her own money as untouchable, not meant to be used to help anyone.

It took an enormous psychological effort for Sue to establish her own bank account, though most of her money still went to the joint account she shared with her husband, Dale. He was nervous about the process, too; he initially feared she was planning to leave him. But once Sue had sat on her own little nest egg for long enough to make Dale believe she wasn't going to cut and run, the stress in Sue's life and in her marriage decreased dramatically. Within a year, she learned that when a man she loved complained, she could simply say, "I'm sorry to hear that, but I know you'll figure things out." Despite some initial fussing, this actually made her relationships better.

You may be thinking that all this has nothing to do with Sue's case of midlife chub-gut. You may be oh so wrong. Eating compulsively was part and parcel of Sue's deep, reptilian-brain reaction to financial pressure and hidden resentment, to her fear of being bankrupted and her anger at the men she had supported. With her assumptions about men and money unquestioned, her constant fear and frustration still in place, Sue went on dozens of diets that ultimately failed. Only when she faced and changed the behavior issues that were causing ongoing stress—a scary process for everyone in her life—was Sue able to eat a healthier diet and take the tire off her tummy, which, by the way, she did brilliantly.

Now it's your turn to make a lifeline to see what circumstances in your life have accompanied periods of weight gain or loss. This may sound like a daunting task, but it's actually surprisingly easy for weight-conscious people. Even if you were completely oblivious to your weight when you were young and skinny, you'll remember feeling relatively chubby or lean at every major event since you started worrying about weight. For example, with 0 being "not fat at all" and 10 being "fattest I ever got," how fat were you in first grade? (Remember, we're not looking at how much you weighed, since you were obviously growing; we just want to know how overweight you felt on a scale from 0 to 10.) What about fifth grade? Your freshman year in college? The age you were when you first fell in love? Last summer?

See, you really can remember. And by plotting your weight over your lifetime, we can find out how the events of your life correlate with your weight. We'll use that information to mine the unconscious lies that may have driven you to overeat and then to create the lifestyle that will allow you to stay fit permanently.

EXERCISE: PLOTTING YOUR FATNESS LIFELINE

On the following few pages, you'll find a form you'll be using to create a weight lifeline, a visual record of your own fatness or lack thereof, based on your subjective recollection of your life. Remember, we're not looking at your actual weight; we want to know the times when you remember being chubbier or leaner. For one person, "fattest ever" may be 35 pounds overweight; for another, it might mean 300 pounds. That's why your chart can't be usefully compared to anyone else's. Its only purpose is to track your weight fluctuations against other events that were happening when you gained or lost.

STEP 1

Starting with the grid on the following pages, put an x across from the number 0 and above the square that says "birth." This signifies that you were not conscious of being overweight at the moment you emerged from your mother's womb. Then, put in more x's above each of the numbers that represent your age. On page 132 is an example of my fatness lifeline up to age 20.

You can see that I was a fairly lean kid but that I put on weight in early adolescence, lost it suddenly at 17, and hit an all-time high at 20. Now, you plot your fatness (subjectively estimated) in each year of your life. If you're older than 80, you can make another grid to finish—this will give you the idea.

Example: Martha's Fatness Lifeline from Birth to Age 20

	BIRTH	AGE 1	AGE 2	AGE 3	AGE 4	AGE 5	AGE 6	AGE 7	AGE 8	AGE 9
10 (FAT)										
9										
8										
7										
6										
5										
4										x
3									x	
2					x	x	x	x		
1				x						
0 (THIN)	x	x	x							

MY AGE IN YEARS

Your Fatness Lifeline from Birth to Age 20

Rate your fatness level from 0 to 10 in the columns above each age
(0 means not overweight, 10 means fattest ever)

	BIRTH	AGE 1	AGE 2	AGE 3	AGE 4	AGE 5	AGE 6	AGE 7	AGE 8	AGE 9
10 (FAT)										
9										
8										
7										
6										
5										
4										
3										
2										
1										
0 (THIN)										

YOUR AGE IN YEARS

Example: Martha's Fatness Lifeline from Birth to Age 20

										x
		x								
		x			x					
			x						x	
x	x				x					
								x		
							x			
AGE 10	AGE 11	AGE 12	AGE 13	AGE 14	AGE 15	AGE 16	AGE 17	AGE 18	AGE 19	AGE 20

Your Fatness Lifeline from Birth to Age 20

Rate your fatness level from 0 to 10 in the columns above each age
(0 means not overweight, 10 means fattest ever)

AGE 10	AGE 11	AGE 12	AGE 13	AGE 14	AGE 15	AGE 16	AGE 17	AGE 18	AGE 19	AGE 20

Your Fatness Lifeline from Ages 20 to 40

Rate your fatness level from 0 to 10 in the columns above each age

(0 means not overweight, 10 means fattest ever)

	AGE 20	AGE 21	AGE 22	AGE 23	AGE 24	AGE 25	AGE 26	AGE 27	AGE 28	AGE 29
10 (FAT)										
9										
8										
7										
6										
5										
4										
3										
2										
1										
0 (THIN)										

YOUR AGE IN YEARS

Your Fatness Lifeline from Ages 40 to 60

Rate your fatness level from 0 to 10 in the columns above each age

(0 means not overweight, 10 means fattest ever)

	AGE 40	AGE 41	AGE 42	AGE 43	AGE 44	AGE 45	AGE 46	AGE 47	AGE 48	AGE 49
10 (FAT)										
9										
8										
7										
6										
5										
4										
3										
2										
1										
0 (THIN)										

YOUR AGE IN YEARS

Your Fatness Lifeline from Ages 20 to 40

Rate your fatness level from 0 to 10 in the columns above each age

(0 means not overweight, 10 means fattest ever)

AGE 30	AGE 31	AGE 32	AGE 33	AGE 34	AGE 35	AGE 36	AGE 37	AGE 38	AGE 39	AGE 40

Your Fatness Lifeline from Ages 40 to 60

Rate your fatness level from 0 to 10 in the columns above each age

(0 means not overweight, 10 means fattest ever)

AGE 50	AGE 51	AGE 52	AGE 53	AGE 54	AGE 55	AGE 56	AGE 57	AGE 58	AGE 59	AGE 60

Your Fatness Lifeline from Ages 60 to 80

Rate your fatness level from 0 to 10 in the columns above each age
(0 means not overweight, 10 means fattest ever)

	AGE 60	AGE 61	AGE 62	AGE 63	AGE 64	AGE 65	AGE 66	AGE 67	AGE 68	AGE 69
10 (FAT)										
9										
8										
7										
6										
5										
4										
3										
2										
1										
0 (THIN)										

YOUR AGE IN YEARS

STEP 2

Consider the age you were when you felt most overweight. What was going on in other areas of your life? Break it down into categories. At your fattest time, what was happening in terms of your:

A. Love life _____

B. Education _____

C. Job or career_____

D. Friendships _____

E. Finances_____

F. Family of origin _____

G. Medical condition _____

AGE 70	AGE 71	AGE 72	AGE 73	AGE 74	AGE 75	AGE 76	AGE 77	AGE 78	AGE 79	AGE 80

H. Children or pets_____

I. Leisure-time activities _____

J. Living situation (physical environment)_____

STEP 3

Repeat the step above for your second-fattest age ever, then your third. Look for common elements. For example, Jim found that whenever he fell in love, he put on weight. He lost weight after breakups. Doris got heavier whenever she was unemployed. What about you? Note any patterns you've noticed in the space below.

_____

_____

_____

STEP 4

Now consider the age you were when you felt *leanest*, when you were effortlessly thin or lost weight successfully. What was going on in your:

K. Love life _____

L. Education _____

M. Job or career _____

N. Friendships _____

O. Finances _____

P. Family of origin _____

Q. Medical condition _____

R. Children or pets _____

S. Leisure-time activities _____

T. Living situation (physical environment) _____

STEP 5

Repeat the step above for the second thinnest time in your life, then the third thinnest time. What was happening during the times you felt skinny and in control? Again, are there common elements? Did your weight drop whenever you had pets, lived in rainy climates, did creative work? Write a note about any common factors in these situations.

_____

_____

_____

STEP 6

As you review your history, notice if certain thoughts, ideas, or story-lines were especially dominant at times when you gained weight. Question these thoughts. For example, the storyline that dominated me at my heaviest times was, "I have to be an old-fashioned lady, like the ones I knew growing up." I was trying to emulate the June Cleavers of a previous generation when my heart wanted to do what I'm doing right now: writing, learning what makes humans tick, and trying to make a difference in people's lives via a career rather than being solely dedicated to the equally noble (but less work-able for me) roles of wife and mother.

What's a storyline that accompanied your fattest times? Write one below, then write down three reasons the story may not be true or useful.

_____

_____

_____

MOVING INTO PREPARATION

The exercise you just completed will do for you what a little reflection on money and men did for Sue. Even by itself, it can be quite helpful; just see-ing a behavior pattern that correlates to weight gain or loss hints that by changing that pattern, you may create better conditions for being lean. But the changes you'll make in your life to help you slim down go beyond the contemplation stage of change. They may include all sorts of diverse, real-world behaviors. Maybe you, like Sue, need your own bank account. Maybe you'd benefit from spending more time with a certain friend, less time with another. It could be that you'll keep eating compulsively until you quit your job. Where weight loss is concerned, all such changes belong in the third stage of change on the transtheoretical model: preparation.

So, congratulations! With this 4-day win, you've completed a full course in contemplation, gaining skills most dieters never acquire (which is why they never get slender, let alone stay that way). In the stage of preparation, which begins on the following page, you'll learn how to shape your life circumstances into a setting that will hold the jewel of your perfect body. You'll also gather information about your particular regimen for eating less and moving more, ultimately choosing the fitness program that will work best for you.

As you do all this, remember that your contemplation exercises are the necessary foundation for each and every positive change you'll be making. If you feel uncertain, derailed, or demotivated, return to the mind exercises of the contemplative, and you'll find your way back to the way of thinking that will succeed even where countless other weight-loss attempts have failed. Anyone can go straight into the action phase of a weight-loss regimen and white-knuckle their way down to a lower weight. But to make thinness long-lasting and effortless, you have to go through the prep steps you'll find in the next few chapters.

"Lifeline" 4-Day Win

Ridiculously Easy Daily Goal: _Each day for the next 4 days, I'll spend 10 minutes thinking about my weight lifeline, recalling any environmental, emotional, or situational factors that occurred during the times I gained or lost weight. I'll write down any factors that seem significant._

Small Daily Reward: _____

_____

Slightly Larger 4-Day Reward: _____

_____

	Dates of My Current 4-Day Win	**Check Off Completed Days Here**
Day 1:	____ / ____ / ____	_____
Day 2:	____ / ____ / ____	_____
Day 3:	____ / ____ / ____	_____
Day 4:	____ / ____ / ____	_____

If you're already on a weight-loss regimen, remember that the 4-day win will enhance it, not conflict with it. If you know what to do, this program will help you do what you know. Feel free to stay on any weight-loss program while you learn 4-day win skills!

PREPARATION

CHAPTER 18

FAT RAT PARK

IDENTIFYING
YOUR NATURAL ENVIRONMENT

I once worked with a client I'll call Ike, who happened to be in prison at the time. Ike, who was serving a couple of years for drug possession and small-time sales, would go to the warden's office and sit with a chaperone present while he talked to me over a speaker-phone. Before our first session, I braced myself psychologically, expecting that helping someone to cope with prison would be the challenge of my life-coaching career. I was stunningly wrong. Ike didn't want me to help him handle incarceration. The reason he wanted to talk to me was that his sentence was almost up, and he was terrified of *not* being in prison.

"When I'm in here," he told me, "I can't get drugs, I don't have to worry about money pressure, there are no fights with my girlfriend. I have trouble sleeping, but that's about it. Once I'm out . . . well, I just don't want to go back."

"So . . . " I asked him, stalling for time, "what's waiting for you at home?"

"I'll go live with my girlfriend in her trailer. Get a job at the meat-packing plant where my buddy works."

"Do you plan to do anything for fun?"

There was a long silence. Then Ike said, "I guess I'll go to some dog fights."

Ooh, I thought. That sounds fun. Not.

Ike and I talked a couple more times before he was released, when he promptly fell off my radar screen. What time we had together was spent planning how Ike could transform his life, so that it would be as enjoyable and fulfilling as prison.

Ike's great fear was that once he returned to the grind of his life outside the Big House, he'd go back to using drugs. Sadly, I'm fairly certain this came to pass. I know for sure that if you put me in Ike's life, I'd do anything from sniffing glue to gulping Oxycontin to break up the boredom, cope with the frightening people around me, increase my tolerance for squalid living conditions, and generally feel a little better. There are some clients that get away, like the 20-pound trout you caught in 1995, and we life coaches wonder about such clients forever. Though I haven't seen Ike since his release, I think about him whenever I deal with a client whose life seems literally worse than prison.

THE SELF-IMPOSED GULAG

I've met a few overweight people who approximate Mike Myers' portrayal of "Fat Bastard" in the *Austin Powers* movies, but most people with weight issues are just the opposite. They're the archetypal "good girls" and "good boys." They're perfectionists and hard workers, eager to please, quick to volunteer for difficult jobs. They serve others extravagantly, while depriving themselves in many ways, food being only one. During the brief periods when they're able to force themselves to live as they think they "should," their lives are so joyless they might as well be living on a gulag.

Take, for example, my client Yvonne, who was always on a diet, but short-circuited her weight loss by bingeing every 3 or 4 days. When I asked her to describe how she'd live on a "virtuous" day, Yvonne described a scenario that made prison sound like a Carnivale Cruise. Ideally, she said, she'd get up before dawn, jog for an hour with the family dogs, fix breakfast for her family, take freshly laundered and selected clothing to each of her children, haul them out of bed, drink a tasteless protein shake while they ate the pancakes and fresh juice she'd prepared, clean the kitchen, make the beds, drive the children to school, and head to her job where she ran an office for a couple of narcissistic plastic-surgery doctors who treated her like a vending machine with breasts. Which they kept telling her she should get lifted.

I don't even want to go on—and we've only gotten to 9 a.m. The rest of Yvonne's "virtuous" day was even worse. There was nothing in the entire schedule she really enjoyed. She never had time to herself. When her inner

Dictator had its way, Yvonne was a captive condemned to hard labor. And she thought she should do the whole thing with a happy spirit and a cheery smile. Small wonder that by her morning coffee break, Yvonne's Wild Child was already sneaking out to a nearby convenience store to stock up on Dots and Cheetos.

Food was serving the same purpose in Yvonne's life that drugs served in Ike's. Both came to me thinking I'd help them enforce better discipline, so that they'd be more obedient prisoners, known for good behavior.

I'm not so big on that.

I like what the Buddha said about enlightenment: wherever you find water, he said, you can tell if it's from the sea because seawater always tastes of salt. And wherever you find enlightenment, in whatever form, you can recognize it because it always tastes of freedom. The taste of freedom, not more rigid compliance, is what Ike and Yvonne both needed. It's what I need if I want to steer clear of overeating. I suspect it's what you need, too. Over-eating is a far more primal, powerful, and inescapable addiction than using artificial chemicals. Fortunately, its allure subsides when the conditions that cause captivity and unhappiness are supplanted by conditions that liberate and nourish the soul.

EXPLANATION: RAT PARK

In the years following the Vietnamese War, a psychologist named Bruce Alexander set out to understand why many veterans who'd taken drugs in Southeast Asia simply stopped using, without much fanfare, after they returned home. At the time, many researchers were doing experiments on lab rats, showing that drugs like heroin and morphine were spectacularly addictive. In labs all over the science-lab world, rodents were being intro-duced to levers that flooded their blood with opiates, and they thumped those levers like hyperactive children playing Whack-a-Mole. Virtually all these rats became hardcore addicts. If they'd had access to tattoo parlors, God knows what their tiny shoulders would have looked like.

After reading many studies of junkie rats, Alexander noticed that all the animals had something in common other than drug addiction. They were all being kept in cages. Now, rats, which have nervous systems a good deal like ours, don't like cages. They like tunnels and burrows, room to roam, and time to spend making friends, appreciating nature, and earning law degrees. So Alexander and his colleagues decided to test the effect of environment on drug use by creating a rodent paradise. They built a zoolike space filled with items and spaces rodents were sure to appreciate. They called this fabulous place Rat Park.

The group then took two groups of rats, one lodged in ordinary cages, the others rambling through Rat Park, and offered them a choice of plain water or sugar-water laced with morphine. The caged rats went for the morphine immediately and were soon acting addicted. The park-dwelling rats, however, preferred plain water. No matter how much sugar Alexander added to the drugged water, the park rats wouldn't drink much of it. Only when he added another drug, Naxolone, which eliminates the intoxicating effects of morphine, did the park rats go for the syrupy morphine-water. In other words, the rats were actively avoiding the effect of the morphine, even though they loved the taste of sugary water. They didn't like getting high.

When Alexander took caged rats, gave them nothing but morphine-water until they were fully addicted to it, and then plunked them in Rat Park and gave them a choice of water that was either pure or laced with morphine, they still decreased their consumption of the drugged water, even though this caused them to go through withdrawal.

I'll bet you a box of Naxolone that the times you gain the most weight are the times you feel trapped and joy-deprived. The next exercise, your first step in the stage of "preparation," will help you identify specific people, places, situations, and activities that either push you toward using food as a mood-lifter or help you feel so free that overeating isn't nearly as tempting.

EXERCISE: RAT TRAP VERSUS RAT PARK RESEARCH

Below you'll find a list of words that describe the feelings you get when you're caught in a cage. In the spaces below the list of words, you'll be instructed to write the names of people, places, activities, and situations that you've associated with these "rat-trap" feelings. Once you've finished that exercise, you'll find a second word list, this one describing the feelings you get when you're in your own special "rat park."

As you see which people, places, activities, or situations trigger trapped or liberated emotions, we'll have a developing picture of what constitutes a rat trap for you versus what comprises your own personal version of rat park.

Rat-Trap Conditions

RAT-TRAP CONDITIONS MAKE YOU FEEL...trapped, deprived, bored, frustrated, smothered, choked, tortured, silenced, hopeless, resentful, starved, worthless, muzzled, confined, forced, hungry, compulsive, uncontrollable, isolated, powerless, suffocated, overwhelmed, imprisoned, dissociated, unproductive, and paralyzed.

Holding these feelings in your mind, WITHOUT JUDGING OR EDITING YOUR OWN RESPONSES, fill in the blanks below.

Three people in my life who catalyze "rat-trap" feelings:

1. _____

2. _____

3. _____

Things these people have in common: _____

_____

_____

Three places in my life that catalyze "rat-trap" feelings:

1. _____

2. _____

3. _____

Things these places have in common: _____

_____

_____

Three activities in my life that catalyze "rat-trap" feelings:

1. _____

2. _____

3. _____

Things these activities have in common: _____

_____

_____

Three situations in my life that catalyze "rat-trap" feelings:

1. _____

2. _____

3. _____

Things these situations have in common: _____

_____

_____

Sunday in Rat Park

RAT-PARK CONDITIONS MAKE YOU FEEL . . . free, satisfied, fascinated, content, absorbed, supported, relaxed, comfortable, heard, confident, grateful, fulfilled, treasured, respected, liberated, calm, secure,
connected, motivated, powerful, expansive, clear, productive, liberated, creative, and flexible.

Again, while holding these feelings in your mind, WITHOUT JUDG-
ING OR EDITING, fill in the blanks below.

Three people in my life who catalyze "rat-park" feelings:

1. _____

2. _____

3. _____

Things these people have in common: _____

_____

_____

Three places in my life that catalyze "rat-park" feelings:

1. _____

2. _____

3. _____

Things these places have in common: _____

_____

_____

Three activities in my life that catalyze "rat-park" feelings:

1. _____

2. _____

3. _____

Things these activities have in common: _____

_____

_____

Three situations in my life that catalyze "rat-park" feelings:

1. _____

2. _____

3. _____

Things these situations have in common: _____

_____

_____

Conditions That Make Me a Fat Rat

Look over the common elements of the people, places, activities, and situations that catalyze rat-trap feelings, and write a summary of them here:

_____

_____

Conditions That Make Me a Skinny Minnie

Look over the common elements of the people, places, activities, and situations that catalyze rat-park feelings, and write a summary of them here:

_____

_____

Since we're still in "research" mode, your 4-day win for this chapter is to sharpen your observational skills and use them to place every significant person, place, activity, and situation in your life in either the "rat-trap" or the "rat-park" category. The next chapter will take you into the "development" part of R&D. You'll start modifying your entire life to eliminate or transform the elements that drive your overeating. You'll do this in little tiny steps, which is what rats always take—and what will most reliably turn you loose in a park of your own design.

"Rat-Park Research" 4-Day Win

Ridiculously Easy Daily Goal: _Each day for the next 4 days, I'll notice and write down one person, place, activity, or event that makes me feel trapped and imprisoned. I'll also note one person, place, activity, or event that makes me feel like I'm home in my natural environment. I'll notice how each of these conditions affects my desire to eat._ _____

Small Daily Reward: _____

_____

Slightly Larger 4-Day Reward: _____

_____

	Dates of My Current 4-Day Win	**Check Off Completed Days Here**
Day 1:	___ / ___ / ___	_____
Day 2:	___ / ___ / ___	_____
Day 3:	___ / ___ / ___	_____
Day 4:	___ / ___ / ___	_____

If you're already on a weight-loss regimen, remember that the 4-day win will enhance it, not conflict with it. If you know what to do, this program will help you do what you know. Feel free to stay on any weight-loss program while you learn 4-day win skills!

CHAPTER 19

THE THREE B'S

BUILDING YOUR OWN RAT PARK

Lola was a veritable encyclopedia of weight-loss knowledge. As a certified dietitian and personal trainer, she knew everything there was to know about eating less and moving more. As a yoga instructor, she was also well-versed in the methods for reaching psychological calm. Yet, between the ages of 36 and 41, Lola had gradually padded on 55 pounds.

Almost as soon as we started working together, we spotted the reason for this: Lola was living a rat-trap existence, locked in by unconscious beliefs about necessity and responsibility. Her wealthy, conservative parents believed that a proper life was one lived in the service of financial security, however grim a task that might be. In fact, the grimmer, the better. Lola had an intensely artistic nature, and to defy her parents—sort of—she'd taken a job as an office manager in the art department of a university. She thought this would be perfect for her Bohemian inner self, but although she could smell paper and turpentine wafting from the studios near her office, Lola routinely spent her time organizing papers and managing employees—both of which she detested.

Since she already knew a lot about fitness, Lola had spent years trying to implement a boot camp–style regimen to peel off fat, tone her muscles, and increase her energy. She bought books on raw-food diets and tried to become a vegan. She signed up for an hour-a-day spin class with a trainer known for enthusiastic brutality. She went on a cleanse that was supposed to be followed by a lifetime of super-healthy diet and exercise control. All of these efforts flamed out like the *Hindenburg*. Lola would sustain her resolutions for a few days and then start chomping her way through pizza and brownies.

Like Lola, most overweight people make the mistake of trying to implement major changes in diet and exercise patterns while ignoring the pressures they're feeling in other areas of their lives. This is like trying to learn meditation while sitting on a hot stove burner. Until the overall conditions of your life are gratifying enough to be enjoyable, you'll have nothing to support better eating and exercise habits, and those habits will never form.

EXPLANATION: LESS IS MORE

Trim tabs are small flaps affixed to the rudder of a seagoing vessel. Even on a huge ship, the trim tabs are practically dainty, sometimes just a few inches wide. To turn a massive boat requires an adjustment to these mini rudders. That changes the flow of water in such a way that the whole rudder can more easily shift its position, catch the current, and ultimately steer the whole shebang. The 4-day wins you've been doing up to now are, in essence, resetting the direction of the trim tabs in your psyche. Now we want to reset the trim tabs for the way you eat and move.

If you tried to turn an ocean liner by turning the large rudder directly, without trim tabs, you'd have to exert so much force that the rudder would probably break off. That's what happens when people try to abruptly and dramatically change their diet and exercise patterns. Eating and moving are two of the most primal components of our behavior, so you can't go from being a fat person to being a thin person without changing virtually everything in your life. Do this suddenly, and you'll waste huge amounts of energy, only to see your new resolutions eventually snap off and sink like stones.

The way to start a fitness program is not this massive "shock and awe" approach. Just as we did with resetting your psychic trim tabs, we're looking for a sneak attack, making tiny changes in little activities that at first might not even seem directly related to food or exercise. Now, I realize you want to lose 10 pounds this week. Again, I give you permission to continue whatever method you think will accomplish this goal. Right now, all your 4-day win requires is that you pick one small aspect of the life situation that makes you feel most like a trapped rat, eliminate that tiny thing from your daily schedule, and replace it with a tiny thing that's part of your ideal rat-park environment.

EXERCISE: THE THREE B'S

Let's start by identifying the thing you hate most about your life on this very day. It might be a person, place, or thing—and I'm not talking about what you're *supposed* to hate, I'm talking about what you *really* hate. Don't be afraid to admit it if your feelings are politically incorrect. Your fatness lifeline will help you spot elements of your life that have a negative effect on you, even if you're supposed to enjoy them. For example, my own weight climbed every time I came close to living a typical homemaker lifestyle. The time I felt most like a rat in a trap was when I had three kids under 5. I loved my preschoolers inexpressibly, but the plain truth was, they bored the crap out of me.

People are horrified when I admit this. You were bored by your *children?* Damn right I was. Chubby cheeks and baby babble are adorable, but I can only sing "Itsy Bitsy Spider" so many times in a single airplane flight and still maintain the will to live. Now my kids are in their teens, and I find them completely delightful, with their smart backtalk and their rude jokes and their friends whose spiky or shaven heads reek of suspicious smoky substances. Teenagers fit right into my rat park, where the rule is "As long as you're under my roof, you will *not* mock an authority system without inviting me to participate!" Few moms I know share my predilections, but if I want to keep from overeating, I have to honor them.

I asked Lola to draw up a to-do list, paying special attention to the things she especially hates. Then I asked her to assign a score from 0 (I'm not the slightest bit peckish) to 10 (I'd like to eat my own head) according to how much thinking of doing each thing made her want to eat. Lola's to-do list, with desire-to-eat scores, looked like this:

EXAMPLE: LOLA'S LIST, WITH DESIRE-TO-EAT SCORES

List of things I plan to do today:	Desire-to-eat score (0 to 10):
Plan fall class schedule	4
Write up schedule	5
Confirm schedule with instructors	10
E-mail schedule to registrar	3

As Lola went through her fatness lifeline and her rat-park testing, it became clear that the administrative details of art school were turning her into a ball of ravenous rage, like Lady Pac-Man. She wanted to eat most when she was dealing with the art-school faculty members. First of all, they tended to be narcissists who treated Lola like chattel. Second, they were all doing what Lola wanted to do—art and teaching—while she did paperwork and administration. Ultimately, Lola quit her job—but that's a big change, one that followed innumerable trim tab alterations.

The first turtle step for Lola, once we'd identified this little nugget of truth, was to choose one of "the three B's." This is how you turn the trim tabs of your life: Focus on a task you hate, and bag it, barter it, or better it. In other words, get rid of it altogether, trade it for something less heinous, or find a way to improve it.

No big deal, right? Wrong.

When you turn a ship 1 degree north, you don't see much immediate change. But when you keep turning it by 1 degree, when the trim tabs kick in and the changes get bigger, you'll find yourself in a very different place after a few days, weeks, years. Lola kept using the three B's at her job for a 4-day win, making just a small alteration every time. A year later, she was happier and more assertive at work, getting ready to jump ship to a new, more creative job—and she'd lost 50 of those 55 extra pounds.

USING THE THREE B'S TO BUILD A BETTER RAT PARK

1. Relax, access the Watcher state, and note your hunger level, from 0 (no hunger) to 10 (starving). Write your hunger score here:

2. Now make a list of "things to do" today. You probably have such a list already. (If you don't have a list already, write one down for today's activities in the spaces you'll find opposite.)

Look at each item on the list, think about doing it, and notice whether you feel an increased need or desire to eat. Put a score by each item, noting how much the thought of it stimulates pseudo-hunger. A score of 0 equals no pseudo-hunger, and 10 means a ravenous feeding frenzy.

Now fill out your list:

List of things I plan to do today: **Desire-to-eat score (0 to 10):**

_____   _____

_____   _____

_____   _____

_____   _____

_____   _____

3. Choosing the most aversive, rat-traplike item on your to-do list, ask yourself the following questions to see where you can apply the three B's:

Can you BAG this activity (avoid the person, place, activity, or situation that is causing the pseudo-hunger) without creating outright catastrophe?

Can you BARTER this activity, by trading or delegating some or all of the elements that are causing pseudo-hunger? Who needs something you can give or a service you could render in exchange for doing the thing you most dislike?

Can you BETTER this activity by adding elements that create your own version of rat park? Can you putter in the garden while talking to your sick mother or play an interesting book-on-tape during your long commute? Think, reader! Think!

Ideas for bagging, bartering, or bettering this activity:

_____

_____

_____

4. If you believe there's nothing you can do to bag, barter, or better your worst responsibilities, you're fibbing to yourself again (not deliberately, I know, but still). Tsk, tsk! Go back to Chapter 12 and review the steps for busting up your fathead thoughts and regaining an open mind.

5. Make one small change in the activity you hate most, replacing a rat-trap condition with a rat-park element.

Lola credits this exercise with helping her stop using food like a pain-killer, because by using it, she ultimately removed much of the frustration that made painkilling necessary. When it comes to building your own rat park, trying to make huge changes results in huge failures, while making a series of smaller changes will ultimately mean there's less of you to change. Try the following 4-day win, bagging, bartering, or bettering whatever you hate most about your daily schedule.

"Use the Three B's" 4-Day Win

Ridiculously Easy Daily Goal: *Each day for the next 4 days, I'll bag, barter,*

or better something on my to-do list that increases my desire to eat.

Small Daily Reward: _____

_____

Slightly Larger 4-Day Reward: _____

_____

	Dates of My Current 4-Day Win	**Check Off Completed Days Here**
Day 1:	_____ / ___ / _____	_____
Day 2:	_____ / ___ / _____	_____
Day 3:	_____ / ___ / _____	_____
Day 4:	_____ / ___ / _____	_____

If you're already on a weight-loss regimen, remember that the 4-day win will enhance it, not conflict with it. If you know what to do, this program will help you do what you know. Feel free to stay on any weight-loss program while you learn 4-day win skills!

CHAPTER 20

FAT IS
A SOCIAL DISEASE

GETTING SUPPORT
FOR YOUR NEW LIFE

Adriana gained 60 pounds during her first pregnancy, and only 15 of them left Adriana's body along with her baby. Her husband, Jeff, complained about this, though he also told her that he was a loyal man who'd stand by her in her fatitude. When her baby turned 3 and went to preschool, Adriana started exercising, cut out junk food, and lost half her excess weight in 6 months. At this point, Jeff began accusing her of infidelity. He knew, apparently through recently acquired psychic powers, that Adriana had carnal intentions toward everyone from the next-door neighbor to Regis Philbin. This upset Adriana so much that she started hitting the nachos and regained 20 pounds. Jeff stopped talking like Othello and went back to his usual "I love you even though you're fat."

Harriet came from a huge family—not a lot of relatives, just huge ones. Like her parents, siblings, and cousins, Harriet had been overweight since childhood. Tragically, when she was 67, Harriet developed Alzheimer's disease. Many Alzheimer's patients experience personality changes, and one of the first changes in Harriet was that she no longer cared *at all* about what anyone thought of her. She suddenly stopped joining her family in their customary overeating and began walking a lot. At family picnics, she'd be the one who ate just a few barbecued ribs before wandering off to smell the flowers. Ironically, in the last years of her life, Harriet was by far the most cardiovascularly fit member of her family.

At age 40, Paula swore she'd do anything to lose weight: give up all delicious foods, work out every day, even have gastric bypass surgery. When she did the rat trap, rat park 4-day win, we found that Paula's overeating skyrocketed during the several hours per day she spent—resentfully, I might add—with her 56-year-old mother. As preparation for weight loss, I suggested that Paula limit an errand-running episode with Mom to 3 hours. This seemed to me like plenty of time to mail some letters and catch up on events that had occurred in the 12 hours the two women had been apart. Apparently, I was wrong. The very thought of a 3-hour limit—and the tizzy into which it would throw her mother—sent Paula into a panic attack. "I'll just stay fat! I'll just stay fat!" Paula told me.

And she did.

My point is that for many of us, the stress factors that drive our weight gain are primarily social. They come from our family interactions, our colleagues, our loves, our losses, and our loneliness. Most animals seek a safe place when they're scared; primates—especially humans—seek a safe *person*. We fear snakes and sharks and grizzly bears, but the beasties that are by far the most likely to harm us are other people. We can be so distraught over words—mere sounds coming from someone else's mouth—that we'll take our own lives. That's why I say fat is a social disease and why building and living in your own rat park requires some special attention to managing your relationships.

EXPLANATION: CHANGEBACK ATTACKS

Given how much suffering comes from social interaction, Sartre may have been right when he famously said, "Hell is other people." Then again, I also agree with Milton's claim, "The mind is its own place, and in itself, can make a Heav'n of Hell, a Hell of Heav'n." Though other people can indeed make our lives difficult, the many woes of interhuman relationships are similar to every other stressor in that they only drive us to overeating when we lie to ourselves about them (unconsciously, of course). Learned helplessness is strongest when it has to do with social interaction.

Dr. Ronald Ruden, a neurologist who studies behaviors such as overeating, says that we can develop a "craving brain" when we believe we're facing "inescapable stress." Pay attention to the times you think "I have to . . ." and "I can't . . ." even though these statements aren't literally true (see Chapters

11 and 12). These phrases are descriptions of inescapable stress, and you'll find that in most if not all of the cases, your feelings of entrapment stem from social pressures. While the truth is that you're less trapped than you think, it's true that your social system is geared to stay as it is. In other words, the important people in your life have helped make you the person you are, and when you begin to change—the goal of the preparation stage—the whole system will be affected. Even the people who criticize your weight may not like it when you upset the apple cart.

A therapist friend of mine uses the phrase "changeback attack" to describe the social pressures we all experience when we make significant transformations in our lives. Adriana ran into a changeback attack when she lost weight and her husband became psychotically jealous (despite the fact that he complained about her being fat). Harriet became impervious to changeback attacks because of her brain disease, so she began eating and exercising according to her body's real needs and tendencies. Paula would do anything at all to lose weight—except set limits on the dreaded outings with her mother and deal with the changeback attack that was sure to follow.

If you're overweight, it's highly likely that the people around you either pressure you to do something you hate or forfeit something you need. As for who, precisely, are your bêtes noirs and how to understand your relationships with these people, well, these are wonderful subjects to discuss with your therapist. This book is about losing weight given your present reality, and that usually doesn't require delving deeply into your childhood. I just want you to notice which interactions with which people seem to correlate with your gaining weight. Conversely, notice any people or social situations that seem to support a healthy, frisky, appetite-controlled version of you. Then we'll modify your social calendar, 4 days at a time, to make your life less and less like prison and more and more like rat park.

EXERCISE: SLENDERIZING YOUR SOCIAL SETTING

Psychologists have labeled two types of change that have very different effects: first-order change and second-order change. First-order change consists of doing more or less of something that's already customary (for example, eating more or less, gaining or losing weight). This kind of change is always reversible. A second-order change involves doing something new and different that's virtually impossible to reverse (going through puberty). One of the reasons people regain weight is that they only make first-order changes, and their social environments don't change at all. Since people and social groups don't like change, and since first-order changes are so easily reversed, the likelihood of being subtly pressured back into old habits is extremely high.

The best way to make a transition that will keep you thin is to create second-order lifestyle changes that are difficult to reverse because of social pressure. You want to decrease your interactions and commitments with people who make you feel trapped, unhappy, and ravenous and increase your interactions and commitments with people who help you stay healthy. Alcoholics Anonymous works partly by providing alcoholics with a ready-made social circle, where they simply spend time around folks who want them to stay sober. Less time with the old social set, more time with these new, supportive people. It's not the whole answer to living a healthier life, but it goes a long, long way.

Look back over the lifeline exercise you completed for Chapter 17 (you did complete it, I assume?) and your rat-trap findings in Chapter 18. Pay special attention to the *people* and *social situations* that seem to be associated with feeling trapped and/or gaining weight. Notice that one such situation may be loneliness, the absence of loving people, rather than the presence of annoying ones. Then survey the people who've been around you at times in your life when you felt energetic and either stopped gaining weight or actually got thinner.

Now we're going to divide the people you interact with into—guess how many?—four categories. In the box on page 166, you'll write down the names of people who support your overweight self and people who will help you get and stay lean. I've labeled these categories as:

1. People who make you want to eat more (we'll call these folks the Munch Bunch)
2. People who make you want to move less (these people are the No-Go's)
3. People who make you want to eat less (the Slender Befrienders)
4. People who make you feel energetic and/or move around more (the Go-Go's)

Note that one person may be in more than one category—in fact, the Munch Bunch and the No-Go's may be the same people. Ditto for the Slender Befrienders and the Go-Go's.

As you list names in the four categories below, remember that people who *tell you* you should eat less and move more are not necessarily Slender Befrienders or Go-Go's—remember Adriana and her "supportive" husband who was actually unconsciously pressuring her to be overweight? The people who belong in those categories are those who actually make you *want to* eat less and become more active.

My Munch Bunch	My No-Go's	My Slender Befrienders	My Go-Go's
————	————	————	————
————	————	————	————
————	————	————	————
————	————	————	————
————	————	————	————
————	————	————	————
————	————	————	————

Your 4-day win for this chapter calls for you to reduce the amount of time, attention, and energy you spend with the Munch Bunch and the No-Go's. You're not going to do this all at once. You're just going to begin edging away from social fat traps. *However, this will be only a first-order change unless you gradually fill in your schedule with people and social situations where you feel freer and get social support for losing weight.*

"But," you may be saying, "I live alone in a refrigerator box under the viaduct. I have no Slender Befrienders or Go-Go's." Be patient; we'll talk about ways you can get more of these people in your life once we reach the action stage of the change process. For now, try these steps for optimizing your social calendar:

1. Pick a Problem Person and Change the Rules

Choose one of your Munch Bunch or No-Go people who really makes you feel and act like a fat, lazy blob. Imagine sitting across a table from this person, having one of your usual chats. Call up the memory of your No-Go as vividly as possible. Now imagine telling this person, "I'm not going to spend as much time with you anymore, and when we're together, I plan to eat a lot less and move around a lot more."

2. Observe the Response

Of course, the person might give you a politically correct answer ("Good, fine. Whatever you want."). But you know in your gut what subtle or overt signals he or she will send telling you that this is a bad change, a violation of your relationship rules, a perversion of the way things should be. This is one more place where the most important weight-loss skill in the history of the universe is necessary, as the next step will remind you.

3. Go to Your Place of Peace

Get calm, breathe, and watch yourself react to the other person's emotional pressure, to the sense of dissonance that may have arisen between you. Sit still, watch the interaction, and breathe until you can *stay calm while the other person tries to pressure you.*

4. Love without Needing to Be Loved

Imagine, as you sit there atop this emotional powder keg, that you have absolutely no need for this No-Go person's love, appreciation, or approval (I'm borrowing this technique from author Byron Katie, who has excellent advice for staying in a fearless, relaxed, and loving state of mind). This doesn't mean you can't love, appreciate, and approve of this person—in fact, loving others is far easier this way. It just means that you're absolutely fine without his or her acceptance.

"But I *do* need their acceptance!" you may be thinking. That thought, that innocent lie, is one of the main reasons you have a weight problem. If, God forbid, something happened to this person, you'd go on. You'd love again. You'd be really sad for a while, and then you'd be fine. The liberating truth is that you don't absolutely have to have love, approval, and appreciation from any specific human being to continue existing. And knowing that you don't need this, oddly enough, will make you much more accepting, more able to receive whatever a specific person has to offer you. Detachment—not grasping at others' love—is the root of genuinely loving relationships.

If you can reach the peaceful and compassionate Watcher within you and see your loved (or hated) ones from this perspective, you'll notice that once again you will become freer to eat or not eat according to your body's needs. You'll feel that subtle but powerful change that lets you off all the hooks pulling you toward obesity. The social hook—the influence of all the relationships in your life—is almost always the most tenacious. The following 4-day win will help you learn to stay peaceful and unattached to the social pressures that have made you overeat.

"Optimizing Your Social Calendar" 4-Day Win

Ridiculously Easy Daily Goal: _Each day for the next 4 days, I'll picture myself telling Munch Bunch and No-Go people that I'm changing the rules of our relationship. I'll observe their responses and practice going to my place of thinner peace even when there is uncomfortable emotional pressure coming from them. I'll do this until I can feel relaxed while imagining their unhappiness._

Small Daily Reward: _____

_____

Slightly Larger 4-Day Reward: _____

_____

	Dates of My Current 4-Day Win	**Check Off Completed Days Here**
Day 1:	____ / ____ / ____	_____
Day 2:	____ / ____ / ____	_____
Day 3:	____ / ____ / ____	_____
Day 4:	____ / ____ / ____	_____

If you're already on a weight-loss regimen, remember that the 4-day win will enhance it, not conflict with it. If you know what to do, this program will help you do what you know. Feel free to stay on any weight-loss program while you learn 4-day win skills!

CHAPTER 21

EAT WHATEVER THE HELL YOU WANT

PREPARING TO EAT LESS

This is another chapter you have already read if you're on the Jump-Start plan. Try taking the quiz again to see if your ideal diet-program needs have changed. Forward!

Derek, an orthopedic surgeon, got out of the shower one morning and noticed he was 80 pounds overweight. "I'd been ignoring it, rationalizing it, hiding it from myself," he told me later. "But that day I just looked at myself and thought, 'Holy crap, I'm fat!'" Derek had never dieted before, so he went out and got himself a weight-loss book: *The Zone Diet*. "It looked pretty reasonable to me," he said, "and it worked." That's all Derek ever needed. Now he's an Ironman triathlete, lean and chiseled as a greyhound. Once he came out of pre-contemplation, Derek needed very little information or structure to get fit and stay that way.

Sharon's weight vacillates by about 25 pounds. When it goes up, she vows to eat less and move more, but on her own, it never really tracks. So she goes to Jenny Craig, where food is provided and she has weekly counseling sessions with a well-trained personal consultant who keeps track of calories so Sharon doesn't have to. This gives her enough structure to feel luxuriously cared for. She enrolls every 5 years or so and thinks of her Jenny Craig experiences as "a vacation from having to deal with my weight all by myself."

Anita is the vice president of a fairly large corporation. Her gift for leadership has made her plenty of money, and her quick mind has absorbed enormous amounts of knowledge. However, having two alcoholic parents left Anita with many emotional-eating tendencies, which used to make her weight zoom up and down like a stoned X Games snowboarder. She tried enrolling in Overeaters Anonymous, going on a medically supervised diet, and even hired her own health-food chef and personal trainer. These strategies always backfired when Anita came to see her support people as authority figures—just like her boozing parents. She'd become angry at the support people, just as she was angry at her parents, then violate the rules they'd set for her. Ultimately, she'd fire them.

As Anita worked with me, she realized that each time her Wild Child gulped a Twinkie or skipped an exercise session, she felt she'd finally triumphed over her parents. But she also felt like the fat kid who deserved her parents' neglect. The fix was for Anita to get out of EASY diet mind (making an external authority the expert) and into CALM mind (learning so much that she became the expert herself). She began reading up-to-the-minute diet research, then designed her own diet and exercise program. She still works with a chef and a trainer, but *she tells them what the program will be, not the other way around.* For someone with Anita's personality and psychological history, the combination of high structure and high information did the trick. She's lost 50 pounds and says she feels great.

I started dieting when I was 6. For the next 30 years or so, my choices about what, when, where, and how much to eat came from my brain, not my body—or anyway, that was the plan. I'd learn what the current expert had to say, memorize calorie counts, then obtain all the chard or trout or bird seed or whatever else was allowed on that program. I'd restrict my eating to the times, places, amounts, and exact food combinations advised by the diet. All would go well until the polar bear effect would kick in and I'd binge my brains out on precisely the foods that were *dis*allowed by my diet du jour.

This process made me a walking calorie calculator. I can tell you the nutritional content of pretty much any food you throw at me (and you'll find that if you constantly tell people the nutritional value of what they're eating, they throw food at you quite a lot). However, I'm also allergic to intellectually based dietary restriction. Three decades of Dictator dominance turned my Wild Child into a rebel with a very clear cause: to eat whatever anyone, including my own mind, instructed me not to eat. Tell me, for example, that I can't have Ho-Ho's, and though I've never partaken of that particular delicacy, I will instantly become a Ho-Ho ho. Forbid carbs, and I'll put away a loaf of bread before you finish talking. Tell me to cut out fat, and I'll butter everything I swallow, including prescription medication.

So these days, I don't follow any diet program. I literally can't. I eat strictly according to appetite: whenever and whatever the hell I want. *But I do this from the position of my inner Watcher,* who isn't compulsive about food and isn't tempted by empty calories or excessive fullness. My one dietary discipline is to return, return, return to identification with your Watcher self and eat only in that state of mind. Ultimately, you'll be able to do this, too, with a high level of confidence that your real nature will choose to eat exactly what's right for you.

When I first gave up on dieting, my famine-damaged brain gravitated toward all the junk food I'd been telling myself not to eat. Gradually, as my brain healed, my Watcher self began asking me to eat healthy food, particularly fruit and veggies. But I always wanted nuts with the fruit and oily dressings or sauces on vegetables. Until recently, I thought I was being a little naughty with the high-fat condiments. But then I read a new study that found oil is necessary to metabolize the beneficial elements of plant foods, increasing the absorption of antioxidants by a factor of 6 or 7. When I read this, I raised my fist in rebel's triumph. It turns out those food combinations appeal to me for good reasons, *reasons my body knew well before my brain.*

This is not to say that I'm a flawless eater or that if you just start frolicking naked through fields of extra-virgin wilted organic arugula, you'll never want to consume anything unwholesome for the rest of your life. Please. What I am saying is that if you become a contemplative, learning to eat according to your body's real appetites without the distortions of mental dietary restriction, you'll find that there's a wisdom in your cells far greater than all the vast sea of information scientists have amassed trying to figure out what diet is best for you.

KNOWING WHAT TO EAT: INFORMATION AND STRUCTURE

The Beck Diet (aka Eating Whatever the Hell You Want) works only if you have fully connected with your Watcher self and *made that self the sole author of your choices.* The truth, as people like Jesus and Rumi and Lao Tzu were always trying to explain, is within us. The Buddha, for example, tried living according to the rules of the rich, which made him fat, and then following the rules of the ascetics, which made him so thin you could throw him across the Indian Ocean by the leg. Finally he decided to toss out the rule-book and refer to nothing but his true nature, and for the rest of his life, he was apparently a middleweight on the Middle Way, healthy, vigorous, and vibrant into old age. As I'm sure Jesus would've been, if they hadn't nailed him to a tree for having the audacity to say that the truth is within us.

So I'd love it if you decided to spend several months just learning to access your Watcher-self, allowing your diet to gradually become healthier, as mine did. But I am also an impatient person, and I realize that you have that event to attend this weekend and then that other event in 3 weeks, and you *absolutely have to be thinner by then.* So you'll probably want to start eating less right now, according to some set of dietary rules you can learn and follow. I view all such programs as crutches—the only diet skill you'll ultimately need is the ability to sustain, or return to, a state of inner peace—but there's nothing wrong with using crutches if you're wounded. If you're a typical dieter, you're as wounded as wounded can be. So let's find out what kind of diet program will work best for you, starting right here and now.

If you're a Jump-Starter, you've already done the drill below—and welcome back. If you've been taking the more scenic route to weight loss, here's how you'll decide what rubber should meet the road.

EXPLANATION: HOW TO CHOOSE A FITNESS PROGRAM WHILE YOUR BRAIN HEALS

There are two components that determine whether a fitness program will work for you: information and social structure. Different weight losers, at different points in their lives, need different levels of each component. If you have tons and tons of nutrition information between your ears, as I did by the time I was an adult, you already have a pretty darn good idea what you should eat to lose weight. You've probably been on diets that made you sick and others that made you feel and look healthier, right up to the point where you lost all vestiges of self-control. You know what combination and amount of food works as a weight-loss program for you.

On the other hand, if you're new to dieting, you'll need to learn some basic information, which you can get from innumerable books, magazines, Web sites, and experts. I'll recommend a few in the following chapter, after we've determined your diet profile. But remember this crucial point: When you turn to any external source for diet information, the goal is to internalize the information so that you can make smart choices, not to see the external source as the author of your decisions. You can get fly-fishing instructions or information on postage stamps without putting your teacher on a pedestal, and the same is true of weight loss. Your ultimate goal is to become the expert who decides what you eat.

Besides information, you may also need an external social structure (one or more people working with you) to support you in applying all that useful diet information. We've talked a bit about limiting your time with the Munch Bunch and the No-Go's and getting more involved with the Slender Befrienders and Go-Go's. This helps your whole life become a fitness-friendly social structure. But something more formal and targeted may be necessary for you as you start losing weight. Some people are naturally comfortable with high levels of structure. They easily and happily adapt to, say, attending weight-loss support groups or having a nutritionist choose, prepare, and deliver their food every day. This gives them the feeling of being cared for, maybe even pampered (it would give me a feeling of violent rage). There's no right or wrong way to feel about structure, but it's important that, at any given point on your journey toward permanent skinniness, you stay embedded in the kind of structure that works best for you.

I'm going to restate the key fact I just told you to remember about information, because it can't be overemphasized: If you choose a highly structured weight-loss program, remember that participating in this structure is your free choice. Never see yourself as the servant of the structure. See yourself as allowing it to serve you.

For example, I had one client, Maureen, who got her weight under control by attending Overeaters Anonymous. She was a rabid True Believer, who constantly referred to OA's rules and regulations. She saw herself as "obeying" the structure and having no personal volition. There was an almost cultlike quality to her devotion. After a few months of this, her Wild Child took over, trying to help her grow up and achieve psychological independence. She began bingeing, then punishing herself for being bad. She was caught in a childlike role, seeing her program as a parent figure: "Do your chores, little girl, and you'll get your reward." On the other hand, I've had several clients who decided to let OA work for them ("I'm a grown-up, but I need company and information") with impressive success.

If you do feel a need for some structure to help you learn to eat better, that's fine, *as long as you observe this need from the position of the inner Watcher.* You'll be an Apprentice, with the open-mindedness and teachable curiosity of a child but without an infant's sense of helplessness or total dependency. Ultimately, we separate from even the most benevolent and well-advised structure, internalizing the set of rules that works best for us. This rise from Apprentice to expert is necessary for permanent weight loss, but it could take years. That's okay. There's no rush.

As you internalize information and gain confidence from structured systems, you'll be like a child learning to walk. You'll fall occasionally. Then you can check with the system to figure out why. You'll implement the methods they advise and *accept or reject all strategies depending on whether or not they resonate with your sense of what is working for your body, mind, and heart.* All information and structure, including the words you're reading now, are meant to help you find your balance and walk on your own. You can. You will. And at that point, you won't need either information or structure as crutches. You'll still be able to learn from them, but you won't depend on them.

EXERCISE: DETERMINING YOUR CURRENT DIET PROFILE

Depending on your personality and past experience, you'll fall into one of four categories in choosing a diet and exercise program. The quiz below will help determine where you fit right now in the structure/information matrix. There are no right or wrong answers, and your responses may well change as the weeks, months, or years go by. Just be honest now so that you can steer toward the best way to lose weight by the time that event comes along, in just 3 weeks.

QUIZ: What's Your Diet Profile?

Answer the following true-false questions as honestly as possible. There is no wrong answer to any of the questions.

1. TRUE   FALSE   I'm not confident enough to be a real do-it-yourselfer; I'm very happy leaving difficult jobs to the experts.

2. TRUE   FALSE   It's hard for me to face a difficult task without support from someone knowledgeable and kind, who can give me feedback and encouragement.

3. TRUE   FALSE   When it comes to learning a new skill, I'd prefer to work with a flesh-and-blood instructor or teacher as opposed to a book or instructional video.

4. TRUE   FALSE   No matter what I'm undertaking, I feel safer and more motivated when I have someone to coach me through unfamiliar tasks.

5. TRUE   FALSE   I don't want to have to keep track of things like calories, fat grams, minutes of exercise, and so on. I have too many things on my mind as it is.

6. TRUE   FALSE   I like working with people, but I also like to know why they do what they do. When I go to the doctor, get my car fixed, or hire a repair person to work on my home, I want to know exactly what he or she is doing and why.

7. TRUE   FALSE   I don't like to work alone, and I don't like being a subordinate. I generally work in teams where I'm the one who really understands what needs to be done and how the team should function.

8. TRUE   FALSE   I'm a natural-born leader. I like taking charge, because I usually understand what's going on better than the people around me.

9. TRUE   FALSE   If money were no object, I'd much rather pay someone to give me a pedicure, do my hair, or

decorate my living space than do the work myself—but I want to make all the decisions about how the job gets done.

10. TRUE   FALSE   I don't have time or patience to perform everyday, routine tasks; I prefer to hire help or delegate the labor for these tasks so I can focus on more interesting challenges.

11. TRUE   FALSE   I love figuring out complicated things on my own. I want to know how everything works, and I get impatient unless I get to direct my own learning process.

12. TRUE   FALSE   It's frustrating for me to work in teams; when I'm trying to achieve a goal, I'd rather go at my own pace than have to coordinate with other people.

13. TRUE   FALSE   I love to get information (from books, experts, TV shows, any source) that explains how the world works in detail.

14. TRUE   FALSE   When I'm passionate about a subject, nothing can stop me from learning everything there is to know about it. I'm almost obsessive.

15. TRUE   FALSE   If you gave me a choice between having an expert do something for me and learning to do it myself, I'd almost always choose the do-it-myself option.

16. TRUE   FALSE   I'm highly self-motivated, and I don't need to know every detail about whatever I'm attempting. Just tell me some basic rules, leave me alone, and let me work!

17. TRUE   FALSE   I like simple, clear goals, and left to my own devices, I'll attain them. Having to involve other people in any effort frustrates me.

18. TRUE   FALSE   I like functioning in systems where there's an established way to do things (for example: the school system, a company, a family tradition, the military). I've earned individual recognition for excelling in such environments.

19. TRUE   FALSE   Give me a job, and I'll get it done if you stay out of my way. Period.

20. TRUE   FALSE   If I believe in what I'm doing, I go straight into action without waiting for anyone else to come along, and I don't stop until I've achieved my objectives.

Scoring

If most of your True responses showed up in questions 1 through 5, you fit what I call the Apprentice profile. You need high structural support but not all that much detailed information. Sharon, the Jenny Craig dieter, is an Apprentice.

If your True answers clustered in questions 6 through 10, you fit the profile of a VIP. You learn a lot about what you want to accomplish, then coordinate people to implement strategies you design. Anita, the CEO with the alky parents, is a VIP dieter.

Getting a lot of True responses on questions 11 through 15 means you have a Scholar profile. High information, not much structure. After my years of diet insanity, I ended up a diet Scholar.

Finally, if you got a lot of True answers on questions 16 through 20, you're an Explorer. You need a few good instructions, a lot of space, and a clear goal but little information and little structure.

The chart on the next page will tell you how to go about starting your weight-loss diet, depending on your needs for information and structure at this point in your life.

HIGH NEED FOR INFORMATION

HIGH NEED FOR STRUCTURE

THE VIP ARCHETYPE
(EXAMPLE: ANITA)

How to Proceed:

Get any or all of the books you'll see listed in the "High Need for Information" section. Then, connect to any or all of the systems listed in the "High Need for Structure" section. Sign up for one or more of these systems (you could have both a dietitian and a trainer, for instance), depending on your resources and preferences. Always remain the designer and administrator of your diet plan. Stay in your Watcher-self to continually connect to your power and keep you from backlashing.

HIGH NEED FOR INFORMATION

LOW NEED FOR STRUCTURE

THE SCHOLAR ARCHETYPE
(EXAMPLE: MARTHA)

How to Proceed:

Get any or all of the books you'll see listed in the "High Need for Information" section. Read them, compare the information from different sources, and see what sounds sensible and appealing to you. If you want any structure at all, connect to a "Low Need for Structure" system. Better yet, design your own weight-loss diet. Stay in your Watcher space as you learn, testing every new piece of information against your own logic and knowledge, instead of enslaving yourself to an intellectual idea of righteous eating.

LOW NEED FOR INFORMATION

HIGH NEED FOR STRUCTURE

THE APPRENTICE ARCHETYPE
(EXAMPLE: SHARON)

How to Proceed:

Get ideas from friends, maga-zines, newspaper articles, or TV about a weight-loss program you might like—maybe one of the systems I've listed in the "High Need for Structure" section. Once you've chosen a system, get connected to it right away. Read whatever material is required by your program, but let the system do the work. Do not make the mistake of thinking this condition should last forever. Your Watcher self will tell you that apprenticeship is the path to mastery, and your goal is to internalize and own the rules you are learning from the system.

LOW NEED FOR INFORMATION

LOW NEED FOR STRUCTURE

THE EXPLORER ARCHETYPE
(EXAMPLE: DEREK)

How to Proceed:

Go online, ask trusted friends, or see your doctor to find out which diet books and systems they think would work for you. Any of the books I've listed under "Low Need for Information" could work. Alternatively, you could enlist in one of the "Low Need for Structure" systems, making sure the one you choose feels right. Familiarize yourself with the rules, and get going! Stay connected to the place of Thinner Peace so that you know if something's off kilter—if the system or informa-tion you're relying on may need to be checked, revised, or traded for something better.

SOME RECOMMENDED DIETS
FOR EACH PROFILE

Given the guidelines in the chart on page 179, there are still infinite diet options available to every weight-loss wannabe. I have a few favorites, based on what I've seen recommended by physicians, nutritionists, and medical researchers I respect and what has worked for my clients and myself at different times in my life. Below you'll find some recommendations for books, Web sites, and systems. You can utilize any of them or any other resource as long as they provide a level of information and social support you like.

People who want high information tend to draw their diet strategies from written material, the more detailed, the better. They'd rather not have a lot of face-time with an advisor. People who like lots of structure prefer flesh-and-blood information sources to printed ones. I've included both human and written components in the recommendations below.

BOOKS FOR PEOPLE
WITH HIGH NEED FOR INFORMATION
(VIP'S AND SCHOLARS)

All these books have corresponding Web sites with updated information. Check 'em out when you crave new data. Also, log on to reputable sites like the American Medical Association's nutrition information or the latest news stories on diets (popular media cover really interesting studies, weeding out the less interesting and giving you the hints you need to Google the latest findings).

> *Ultrametabolism,* by Mark Hyman
> *8 Weeks to Optimum Health* and *Eating Well for Optimum Health,* by
>   Andrew Weil, MD
> *The Way to Eat,* by David Katz, MD
> *Eat More, Weigh Less,* by Dean Ornish, MD
> *The South Beach Diet,* by Arthur Agatston, MD
> *The Sonoma Diet,* by Connie Guttersen
> *French Women Don't Get Fat,* by Mireille Guiliano
> *The Zone Diet,* by Barry Sears

Pritikin Program books, by Robert Pritikin

Mediterranean diet (go online to find research from many different authors)

Glycemic Index diet (multiple sources; see Christiane Northrup's online newsletter)

BOOKS FOR PEOPLE WITH LOW NEED FOR INFORMATION (APPRENTICES AND HEROES)

Get one that looks doable, and do it. If you're a Hero, you'll base your diet on the book you choose. If you're an Apprentice, you don't have to read anything; just sign on to a good system and let your advisors teach you to eat well.

Dieting for Dummies, by Jane Kirby, RD

8 Minutes in the Morning, by Jorge Cruise

The South Beach Diet for Beginners, online

Get With the Program, by Bob Greene

Body for Life, by Bill Phillips

Fat Loss 4 Idiots online information resources

SYSTEMS FOR PEOPLE WITH HIGH NEED FOR STRUCTURE (VIP'S AND APPRENTICES)

These are just a few systems that are easy to locate nationwide. Your doctor, local health clinic, or independent weight-loss centers may be good, too. Don't be the system's slave; choose one to *work for you, not vice versa.*

Jenny Craig (the highest-touch, most thoroughly supportive program out there for people who aren't zillionaires but are willing to invest in their health and need systems to do it. I worked with them to develop psychological weight-loss tools because I respect and recommend their services.)

Weight Watchers (not quite as high-touch as Jenny Craig; food available but not required; less expensive but also more work)

Overeaters Anonymous (very rigid structure, lots of personal contact, and it's free!)

Personal chef services (many programs are surprisingly affordable; check the Internet and your Yellow Pages)

eDiets (an excellent service that helps you personalize your plan online; will help you structure an eating program around just about any diet out there; lacks the face-to-face contact with real people that you may need, especially at first)

SYSTEMS FOR PEOPLE WITH LOW NEED FOR STRUCTURE (SCHOLARS AND EXPLORERS)

Try any of these. Or not. Ideally, you'll either design your own program (if you're a Scholar) or pick a decent one and just do it (if you're an Adventurer). Or, you could choose not to use any system at all, just act on what you know.

The Beck Diet (eat whatever the hell you want, but only from a mental place of peace)

Any buddy system (have friends lose weight along with you, or bet a pal you can drop weight)

The Oprah "Spa Girls" plan (read about setting up a weight-loss group on Oprah's Web site)

Online program of your choice (browse at will, pick anything interesting, try it on for size)

SlimFast (buy the shakes, follow the plan)

I have to trust you to use your good sense, knowledge, and instincts when it comes to the latest fad diet du jour. When I was about 12, I tried a diet that recommended eating nothing but cayenne pepper, lemon juice, and maple syrup. At this writing, eons later, I hear this diet is all the rage in New York. "People are losing tons of weight on it!" an excited friend recently told me. Well, of course. People could lose tons of weight by refusing to eat anything except what they can lick off the exhaust pipe of a diesel truck, too. Then they'd get a major case of famine brain, go back to eating normally at best, or (more likely) overeat as a compensation for the toll the diet took on their physiology and psychology. If the Shiny Object of Tomorrow Diet sounds extreme and strange, it is.

So, for your next 4-day win, you'll pick your program, figure out the menu, and stock your house with the necessary supplies. You'll get all braced to start eating less. And you will immediately notice a problem. That problem is that none of the programs you might have chosen is likely to contain an explicit eat-a-brownie-the-size-of-my-head option. Now that you're actually considering starting that program, suddenly that's the only option that seems worth exercising—and you want to exercise it very, very badly.

Not to worry. Just read the next chapter.

"Pick a Diet, Any Diet" 4-Day Win

Ridiculously Easy Daily Goal: _For the next 4 days, I'll spend 10 minutes a day checking out the weight-loss programs listed in this chapter. I'll pick a program, then I'll go on to read Chapters 31 and 32 of this book, so that I can design my first "eat less" 4-day win._ _____

Small Daily Reward: _____

_____

Slightly Larger 4-Day Reward:_____

_____

	Dates of My Current 4-Day Win	**Check Off Completed Days Here**
Day 1:	_____ / _____ / _____	_____
Day 2:	_____ / _____ / _____	_____
Day 3:	_____ / _____ / _____	_____
Day 4:	_____ / _____ / _____	_____

If you're already on a weight-loss regimen, remember that the 4-day win will enhance it, not conflict with it. If you know what to do, this program will help you do what you know. Feel free to stay on any weight-loss program while you learn 4-day win skills!

CHAPTER 22

BURY A BUNCH OF BONES

DEVELOPING ABUNDANCE BRAIN

Some friends of mine adopted a rescue dog named Bonkers who has food issues. The scurvy knaves who abandoned him as a puppy also nearly starved him, so even now, after being well-fed for years, Bonkers apparently feels he shouldn't get too confident about the future. Every day, he gets a special treat—a fake bone made out of some horrifying meat-processing by-product—and every day, he buries it next to his owners' fireplace. The thing is, there's no dirt next to the fireplace, just brick. So Bonkers *pretends* to dig a hole, then puts the bone in the *pretend* hole, and then covers it up with *pretend* dirt.

As long as everyone in the household joins Bonkers in acting as if the bone has been hidden away, all is peaceful. But if some ignorant human picks up the bone or even looks at it in a knowing way—well, that's how Bonkers got his name. He can go from peaceful lapdog to insane survivalist miser in a heartbeat. His owners have decided that rather than spend money on a dog psychologist, they'll just join Bonkers in acting as if he has a secret cache of food that no one can see or disturb. In other words, the entire household lives in deliberate denial, not unlike some presidential administrations. But it seems to be working for them.

In this chapter, we'll see how you can benefit from similar psychological tricks. If you finished the 4-day win in the last chapter, you chose a diet method that fit your profile and found out (either by getting information or signing up for a program) what the recommended menu was. If you're going

185

to start on your diet right now, please jump ahead to Chapter 30, which has specific instructions for limiting food intake without causing famine brain to develop. No matter what diet you've chosen, don't adhere to it so strictly that you feel absolutely famished. Ever. *Allowing yourself to become ravenous and denying yourself forbidden foods will make you fatter.* If you can resist these temptations, proceed full speed ahead. But if you experience these issues, you'll need some ammunition to fight back these urges.

EXPLANATION: COUNTERING FAMINE BRAIN WITH ABUNDANCE BRAIN

If you're following a published fitness program, it probably includes instructions about removing all forbidden, fattening foods from your house. This is one of the most common things I hear from diet advisors. Personally, I've never seen it work.

First of all, removing fattening food from your house to make yourself eat less is about as effective as Prohibition was in making Americans drink less. If we crave unhealthy food (and everyone with famine brain does), we'll get it and eat it. Remember the guys in the Ancel Keys study, who became obsessive bingers after a few months of dieting? They didn't start out fat or binge-prone, though they all had plenty of food available. It was *limiting* their food intake, once they'd gotten good and hungry, that caused them to obsess about forbidden food, to hunt it, hoard it, steal it, and eat up to 10,000 calories of it at a single sitting. Deprivation, not available food, pushes people into famine brain.

DEPRIVATION AND FAMINE BRAIN

Famine conditions cause the brain-body connection to haul out some very big neurochemical guns. The hungrier we get, the more a hormone called dopamine floods an area of our brains called the nucleus accumbens. This causes goal-seeking activity, including the search for food. If we eat immediately, the nucleus accumbens gets swamped with serotonin, we feel satisfied, and we stop thinking about eating. If no food shows up, dopamine levels keep rising, driving increasingly urgent food-seeking. Over time, this creates structural changes in the brain so that cravings come to dominate our thoughts and behavior—even if we get food. For someone who has endured famine, the body may be stuffed, but the brain still signals, "Hungry!"

Just today, my friend Annette (she of the frequent fasting) told me, "My stomach is completely full, and I'm completely ravenous." This is what happened to the men in the Keys study. It's what happened to the fashion model who ate herself to death. It's what happens to people who have gastric bypass surgery but keep eating until they burst their stomachs.

As usual, please note that this makes perfect evolutionary sense. In a wild state, an animal in a famine-stricken area would survive longer if it obsessively focused on finding food. Once it found a food source, it would make sense for the animal to eat as much as possible and bank the excess as fat. In conditions of long-term deprivation, the brain makes sure to motivate exactly that behavior. It doesn't matter whether the deprivation comes from the environment (a real famine) or from the thinking mind (a diet).

I spent years avoiding fattening food to keep myself from overeating, and I developed a case of famine brain that nearly made me suicidal. When I was a college freshman, always on a diet, I'd eat the meager dinner allowed by the regimen I was on. Then, while I wasn't hungry, I'd engineer my environment so I couldn't get more food until the next day. I'd stay away from the student union at the hours when food was available. I'd make sure I had no money, not one red cent, that I could spend on food. Then I'd settle in and try to focus on studying.

As the year went by, I started to experience the full nightmare of a famine-modified brain. I'd lie in bed, exhausted but too hungry to sleep, until 2 or 3 in the morning. Then I'd get up and ransack my dorm room, looking for spare change. When I didn't find it (of course I didn't find it; I'd made sure of that myself), I'd head out into the zero-degree weather and run for hours, desperately checking to see if there were any 24-hour convenience stores giving out food samples or throwing away food that was still packaged. Or not packaged. I'd run almost all night. Usually, I found nothing edible. But when I did, no matter what it was, I ate it. I couldn't *not* eat it. I might as well have tried to stop breathing.

This ghastly ritual took on a life of its own. I began bingeing during the day, regaining some of the weight I'd lost. If I tried to leave the dining hall without eating at least enough calories for a full day, I'd be attacked by indescribably intense fear. After a binge, I was anything but physically hungry, but my famine brain would still awaken in the wee hours, driving me out into the cold on its nightly food search. My own brain felt like a cunning parasitic monster I'd created myself simply by following the advice of a well-meaning diet-book author who advised me to stay away from fattening food.

More than 20 years later, I think my brain is almost back to normal. But remember, famine brain is a structural reality, and I've had to accommodate mine, adjusting for it the way someone with dyslexia has to adjust reading habits. I no longer obsess about fattening food, overeat on fattening food, dream about fattening food. But I *have* fattening food. I have lots and lots of it. In fact, it's only when I don't have it that I feel driven to eat it.

COPING WITH FAMINE BRAIN BY PROVIDING ABUNDANCE, NOT MORE DEPRIVATION

Bonkers the dog is not fat. He has experienced starvation, and he appears to have lots of craving brain symptoms. But he doesn't eat everything he's given; he eats what his tummy wants. He doesn't have to carry extra food on his body because he has cleverly hidden it in the imaginary dirt next to the fireplace. He only obsesses about it when it seems to him that someone is about to take away his secret cache.

Like Bonkers, I lay in serious supplies no matter where I go. I have several boxes of fine chocolate in my house, slices of incredibly rich key-lime pie in the fridge, lots of high-calorie snacks to carry on airplane flights. Once in a blue moon, I'll take a bite of chocolate truffle or pie, notice that it makes me feel kinda gross, and throw the rest away. When I can't reach fattening food (for example, when I forget to take my usual bag of candy on an airplane flight), the ghost of famine brain kicks in. Then and only then, unless I seriously focus on staying mentally balanced, I overeat.

I think that our brains are geared to relax famine responses *when we know we have food stored* even more than when we've gorged ourselves. This is why Bonkers is a calm and happy dog as long as he has his bone safely airburied. Clearly, an instinctive hoarding impulse drives him to do this, since he repeats the behavior even when no actual dirt is available. Take away the stored food, and it only increases the impulse to guard against starvation by eating. When I suggest to Annette that she deal with her brain hunger by assuring herself that she can go to the bakery and get as many cookies as she wants any time, she suddenly doesn't feel ravenous anymore.

The fine folks at See's Candies, where I buy a lot of excellent chocolate I'll never eat, tell me that they used to have a real problem with employees snarfing merchandise—which was strictly forbidden—until they decided to allow them to have as much chocolate as they wanted. Now, new employees tend to eat lots of chocolate for (yup) 3 days. On the fourth day, the new status quo has kicked in, and their brains realize, "Goodness, I'm surrounded by limitless chocolate, and I can have all I want." The workers stop bingeing and level off at about three chocolates a day. One See's worker told me that she binges on other foods but now has no trouble bypassing the chocolate she once craved. "Who wants chocolate?" she said, rolling her eyes. "I'm up to *here* in chocolate."

Many of my clients tell me, "I can't eat that first piece of chocolate/ potato chip/cookie, or I'll never stop." This is dichotomous thinking, and if you have it, you're not in a good psychological position to lose weight. Try the following exercise.

EXERCISE: BURYING BONES FOR ABUNDANCE BRAIN

1. Picture Your Sinful Food

Think of your favorite forbidden food: greasy, salty chips; creamy pudding; fatty filet mignon browned to perfection. Think about how it looks and smells, how it tastes and feels when you munch it. How much would you like to eat?

Question: How many servings did you imagine? Usually, the answer is one. And if you're at all hungry, that one serving of your favorite culinary crime probably has your mouth watering. If you could get at it, you'd eat it and look around for more.

2. Go to the Place of Thinner Peace

Now, take a minute to observe your craving mind, your Wild Child, and the Dictator thoughts that may arise to criticize it. Be kind. Observe. Become the Watcher, taking a seat in the mental place of peace.

3. *Imagine Magical, Limitless Amounts of Your Sinful Food*

Go back to the memory of your forbidden food, only now imagine that instead of one serving, you're sitting at a table groaning with an endless supply. Five hundred steaming pounds of French fries. A thousand cheeseburgers. Ten 5-gallon containers of premium ice cream, chilled and ready to eat indefinitely. And magically, this huge mass of food is going to follow you everywhere for the rest of your life. It won't get in the way of anything. It will just always be *there*. Always, always, always.

How much do you want now?

Usually, this second answer—imagined in a state of endless abundance rather than limitation—actually reflects how physically hungry you are. It's a decision made in a state of plenty, not famine. I do this exercise in real life with clients who claim they can't stop eating a certain food. We go to a place where we can find their sinful food in huge abundance, then think in terms of having this abundance available forever. Confronted by 100 pounds of chocolate, a buffet table of ribs, or 1,000 doughnuts, they switch out of famine brain and ask for moderate servings—or lose interest.

REAL-LIFE OPTION FOR BEGINNERS

If you want to see this work in real life, get together with a friend who can keep you from disappearing into famine brain bingeing. Go to a restaurant and order several servings of your favorite food, much, much more than you want to eat. Your friend is going to keep the food you can't finish, and you can have it later, any time you want it.

Get into your Watcher identity, and start eating. Notice how much food it takes to fill you up. Notice that in a state of infinite supply, you don't want to keep eating past this point.

REAL-LIFE OPTION FOR EXPERIENCED THINNER PEACENIKS

Repeat the beginner's option above, but this time eat until you're satisfied and then save the remaining food for later. You may eat it later, or you may keep it in your refrigerator until it has spent so much time evolving in there that it begins speaking to you in full sentences, at which time you'll throw it away. (If the thought of throwing it away upsets you, just keep reading. We're getting to that.)

I'm going to stop short of saying you should fill your house with candy and other fattening trash foods (though it works for me and Bonkers). I am saying that *if you begin obsessing about a certain kind of food or bingeing uncontrollably with it, you need to actively work on relaxing famine brain by re-establishing conditions of abundance.* Your 4-day win requires that each day you get into your balanced, peaceful Watcher self, buy yourself a generous amount of your favorite food, eat mindfully, stop when you're full, and *remember that you can have more of the same food when you feel hungry again.*

If you have a badly distorted famine brain like mine, this is only the beginning of a long recuperation. But the more you assure yourself that you'll never be cruelly deprived or starved again, the sooner you'll establish a psychological condition that reflects abundance rather than maximizing famine responses to the point of madness. Try the following 4-day win to start the process. Then, in the next chapter, we'll throw it all away. Well, anyway, some of it.

"Burying Bones for Abundance Brain" 4-Day Win

Ridiculously Easy Daily Goal: _Each day for the next 4 days, I'll practice eating some of my forbidden foods, stopping when I'm full, and remembering I can have more of what I want the next time I'm hungry. I'll notice the effect this has on my cravings._ _____

Small Daily Reward: _____

_____

Slightly Larger 4-Day Reward: _____

_____

	Dates of My Current 4-Day Win	Check Off Completed Days Here
Day 1:	___/___/___	_____
Day 2:	___/___/___	_____
Day 3:	___/___/___	_____
Day 4:	___/___/___	_____

If you're already on a weight-loss regimen, remember that the 4-day win will enhance it, not conflict with it. If you know what to do, this program will help you do what you know. Feel free to stay on any weight-loss program while you learn 4-day win skills!

CHAPTER 23

TRASH THE TREASURE, DON'T TREASURE THE TRASH

Mollie's face is contorted with effort. She's breathing hard and sweating as though lifting a minivan or giving birth to a baby that has decided to come out sideways.

Actually, she's trying to discard an Oreo.

Now, Mollie is a powerful, smart, committed, and talented woman. She runs her own successful cattle ranch, doing everything from calf roping to hardball negotiating with suppliers and buyers. But that Oreo has an almost mystical power over her. Although she's hired me specifically to help her lose weight, and though I've told her this is the next step in her preparation phase, and though we're doing this exercise on a closed course with a defibrillator handy, I think Mollie may actually die before she can drop the cookie into the wastebasket.

"I was . . . ," she whispers, "I was . . . brought up . . . not to do this."

True, Mollie's parents were Depression-era farmers who saw wasting food as criminal. But her difficulty with throwing away food has also been reinforced by Mollie's diet history. Obediently cleaning her plate at three meals a day, she became a chubby child and a chubbier woman. Active as she is, the weight of her 5-foot 4-inch body has vacillated between 180 and 210 pounds her whole adult life. She's starved herself repeatedly, and each time her brain has become more and more attuned to famine conditions, more and more likely to crave and consume too much food.

"Drop it, Mollie," I say, trying to be kind but firm and sounding like Cruella DeVil.

She laughs nervously. "Oh," she says, "you mean *today*?" But with one final gasp, she finally drops the Oreo in the wastebasket. Once it's there, she still can't take her eyes off it. She's definitely tempted to exercise the three-second rule and go in after it.

"Let it go, Mollie," I tell her. She raises her eyes from the Oreo and lets out a sigh of surrender. "Excellent," I say. "Good work!"

EXPLANATION: WHEN OPPORTUNITY KNOCKS, LOCK THE DOOR

If you were raised like Mollie (and most people were), one of the biggest obstacles to losing weight is that you have trouble throwing away food. You'll stuff yourself to the eyeballs if that's what it takes to clean your plate. Even more significantly, if you've ever dieted, your brain has become hyper-charged to make you crave and eat rich or sweet foods and resist throwing them away. Despite living in an environment where food is actually so abundant it's an actual public-health threat, your physiology operates as though you're rushing around a forest looking desperately for nonpoisonous mushrooms and gnawing the bark off trees.

You were born, bred, and conditioned to be what biologists call an opportunistic eater. Dogs are opportunistic eaters compelled by scent, which is why my beagle can inhale a family-size pizza one minute and the next minute swear on a stack of Bibles that he's starving, really, really *starving*. Snakes are opportunistic eaters attracted to the heat of warm-blooded animals, which is why the day before I wrote this, a boa constrictor in Ketchum, Idaho, had to undergo surgery after eating—this is true—a queen-size electric blanket. Human bodies are geared to eat opportunistically when we see, smell, or even think about something yummy.

Opportunistic eaters, especially those who have experienced some form of deprivation (dieting), experience intense resistance when it comes to letting tasty items go to waste. Don't let that last brownie just sit there! Don't throw it away! Think of the children starving in the Sudan! News flash: Starving Sudanese children remain stubbornly unrelieved while someone in Des Moines attains the physical dimensions of a walrus. If you want to show your gratitude for the abundance in which you live, start by teaching your brain to accept that abundance. Then go to that internal balance point, the one that allows you to eat exactly as much as your body needs to be its healthiest. (By the way, this is the psychological state likely to motivate you to do something, like donating money, that may actually help starving Third-World children.)

To be a thin person indefinitely, you must reframe your whole perception of wasting food. Food is wasted when a diabetic eats it, gets sicker, and loses a limb. It's wasted when it clogs your arteries, raises your blood pressure, and causes a heart attack or a stroke. If you're swallowing food you don't need, packing it on as fat, every molecule that makes you less healthy rather than more healthy is being wasted.

Beagles and boa constrictors, as far as I can tell, don't have the psychological wherewithal to walk through the logic of this reframing. But as a human, you can logically see why a famine response at a never-ending smorgasbord leads to gluttony, ill health, and obesity. A crucial step in unlocking the patterned responses and cravings that cause you to overeat is learning to discard food when you don't need it. In fact, this is so important in reconfiguring your habitual responses that I suggest you *always* leave food on your plate. If you're really so hungry that you physically need every bit of food in front of you, go get a refill just so you'll have a little something to throw away. Make cleaning your plate seem odd and irregular.

Are you getting anxious, angry, or shocked at this suggestion? If you need to gain weight, that's an appropriate reaction, and I encourage it. If you're actually on the hefty side (and why else would you be reading this?), your negative reaction to throwing away food is a problem. Let me restate this just in case I haven't made myself clear: THROWING AWAY FOOD WHEN YOU'RE TOO FULL TO EAT IT IS NOT WASTEFUL. IT IS WASTEFUL TO EAT THAT FOOD, THEREBY CAUSING YOURSELF TO BECOME A FAT DEAD PERSON.

All right, then. Let's proceed to this chapter's exercise.

EXERCISE: TRASH THE TREASURE INSTEAD OF TREASURING THE TRASH

This next exercise is a skill you might use daily for the rest of your life, possibly at every meal. It may appall the spirits of your perpetually hungry ancestors, but in today's world, it's an essential tool for staying healthy.

Learning to Trash the Treasure

*1. Wait until you're hungry, then get a whole bunch of very righteous
    food.*

By very righteous food I mean something inexpensive and very good for
you, like salad or boiled vegetables. You're choosing inexpensive food so it'll
be less painful to bid farewell to it, as I'm just about to ask you to do. You're
choosing righteous food because it's almost certainly the food choice you
aren't making right now, although you feel you should be, and you don't
find it terribly appealing. Make sure you prepare more food than you really
want to eat. Put a huge serving of the very righteous food on a plate, then sit
down and get ready to eat.

2. Become the peaceful Watcher

Before you eat, center yourself. Tune in to your physical sensations, then
your emotions. Watch your thoughts. Observe what your Wild Child is
thinking and feeling, then what's going on with your inner Dictator. Offer
them both loving thoughts ("May you be well, may you be happy, may you
be free from suffering") until you feel connected to the Watcher. Now turn
your attention to the very righteous food, and observe it from the position of
the Watcher. Strangely enough, you may notice that the food now seems
more appetizing than it did when you first sat down.

*3. Eat some of the very righteous food, watching your own sensations, until
    you're satisfied.*

Notice everything you feel and think as you eat. Spend some time chew-
ing the food, observing its taste, texture, and temperature. Notice how it
feels to swallow and how your stomach reacts once the food reaches it. Rank
your fullness level with every bite, with 0 signifying "hungry" and 10 signifying "stuffed to the gills." Eat this way (it's a common mindfulness meditation) until you feel a sense of physical satiation. You want your hunger level
to get to about an 8—not stuffed, but definitely satisfied.

4. Throw away the remaining very righteous food.

Remain in the place of the Watcher as you throw away the food. Watch
the Dictator freak out: "You're being wasteful!" and marvel that this is the
very same part of you that's always criticizing you for eating too much. See
if your Wild Child feels emotionally starved and abandoned or wants to

keep eating just for eating's sake or becomes desolate over starvation over-seas. From the Watcher's calm perspective, remind all parts of yourself that throwing away this particular excess of righteous food is the most sensible thing you can do. Adopt an orphan, if you must, but learn to see that eating food you don't want is actually less helpful to the world than throwing it away, because it's making *you* less helpful to the world.

5. *Wait until the next time you're hungry, and repeat the whole process with moderately righteous food.*

Once you've learned to throw away cheap, unappealing, or even nasty-tasting food without having a panic attack, push up the stakes by doing this whole exercise with something a little more expensive and tastier—say, oat-meal. Repeat Steps 1 through 4, above. You may have a harder time calming yourself. You may have to adopt two orphans. Do whatever it takes, because you're about to go up a notch.

6. *Wait until the next time you're hungry, and repeat the whole process with moderately wicked food.*

Depending on your tastes and mores, moderately wicked food might be mashed potatoes, presweetened cereal, red meat, scrambled eggs, lasagna . . . see, things are starting to get interesting. Be very careful to eat slowly and remain mindful of your physical sensations while you eat—now that we're talking about wicked food, you're in much more danger of going off the rails and mindlessly stuffing yourself.

It will also be harder to deal with your anxiety about throwing away the food that still remains when your gut hunger is satisfied. It may help to tell your Wild Child that the next time you get hungry, you will get more of this food and eat it again. But continue doing this exercise with moderately wicked food until you can stop eating when satisfied but are not stuffed and throw away the leftovers without panicking.

7. *Wait until the next time you're hungry, and repeat the whole process with extremely wicked food.*

You know what I'm talking about. I'm talking about That Food, the dish you can't stop eating and would never, ever throw away—except that now you're going to stop eating it and throw it away *when you've had enough to satisfy your hunger.* Again, if you find yourself panicking, reassure your

Wild Child that there is plenty of extremely wicked food available and that you can have some more the next time you get hungry.

Remember that, in general, you'll do well to save leftover food and cache it for later. But right now, the emphasis is on learning to leave food uneaten, then throw it away. Even good food. Even tasty, expensive food. Even food your adorable Slavic grandmother whipped up with her own meaty forearms (be discreet, of course—what Grandma doesn't know won't kill her). Try trashing at least some food after every meal for 4 days (the 4-day win on the opposite page) and then make it a habit at every meal.

Getting past the mental block that says, "Don't you leave this table until you've cleaned your plate!" is a stepwise change; once you've gotten over the threshold, you'll be far more able to tune into actual hunger and satiety cues, which will tell you the real amount nature meant you to eat at any given meal. Someday, I hope we will meet to break bread together, then throw it away. Think of me as the coach who sits by your elbow, cheering you on as you throw away food you never wanted. Deciding how many orphans to adopt—well, that's up to you.

"Trash the Treasure" 4-Day Win

Ridiculously Easy Daily Goal: *Each day for the next 4 days, I'll get more food than I want, eat mindfully from the position of the Watcher until I feel satisfied, then throw away the food that's left over.*

Small Daily Reward: _____

_____

Slightly Larger 4-Day Reward: _____

_____

	Dates of My Current 4-Day Win	**Check Off Completed Days Here**
Day 1:	_____ / ___ / _____	_____
Day 2:	_____ / ___ / _____	_____
Day 3:	_____ / ___ / _____	_____
Day 4:	_____ / ___ / _____	_____

If you're already on a weight-loss regimen, remember that the 4-day win will enhance it, not conflict with it. If you know what to do, this program will help you do what you know. Feel free to stay on any weight-loss program while you learn 4-day win skills!

CHAPTER 24

FLAVORS FOR FLOUTING FAMINE BRAIN

WEIRDLY COMPELLING NEW DIET RESEARCH

Once I got to spend a couple of amazing days at a game park in South Africa. Hunting has been banned in this area for more than a century, so the animals who live there have no fear of humans. Our camp had a large, open-air deck where we'd have afternoon tea (the traditions were all very British) while overlooking a waterhole populated by gamboling hippopotami and thirsty antelope. Each table on the deck had the usual European condiments—butter, sugar, salt, pepper. These had to be kept covered with heavy ceramic lids. Otherwise, vervet monkeys would rush in, grab the butter and sugar, take it down to the river, mix it together, and eat it.

Yup, that's right. Monkeys—untrained, wild monkeys—cook.

The reason they do this, which is still not completely understood by science, can make weight loss and maintenance dramatically easier for you.

Here's the question: Why do the monkeys go to the trouble of blending the butter and sugar together instead of just eating each food separately? You know the answer: Because eating large quantities of these foods independently—say, a whole stick of butter followed by a whole cup of powdered sugar—is disgusting. The taste and texture would make you want to puke. But combine straight powdered sugar and straight butter, and what do you have? Buttercream candy or cake frosting, which many of us can eat until the cows come home, at which point we milk them to get more butter.

Foods are more palatable when they are made up of combined flavors and textures, because we need different food elements to survive. As I mentioned in my reference to oily vegetables (see last chapter), Mother Nature has designed us to be most pleased by the combination of vitamins, minerals, proteins, fats, and sugars we need to be healthy. Unfortunately, Mother Nature has not been taking our calls lately, and she still thinks we live like vervet monkeys, riding the edge of starvation and moving around all day long in search of scarce calories. So we, like the monkeys, are powerfully drawn to food combinations such butter and sugar, which put as much fat on our asses as Mother Nature, who is basically a coldhearted bitch, can arrange.

EXPLANATION: TASTE AND TUBBINESS

The sense that's most attuned to food combinations, obviously, is taste. That's why the whole complex process of food consumption, digestion, and allocation takes its cues from flavor. Until recently, no one even suspected that the taste of the foods we eat has a strong, direct link to how much we weigh. A calorie was a calorie, scientists assumed. A gram of fat was a gram of fat. How they tasted made no difference. Well, nutrition specialists are now finding that these assumptions were in error. All kinds of odd research findings are beginning to show that flavor matters a lot in weight loss and maintenance.

For example, rats that eat a certain amount of dry bread ingredients put on less weight than rats who eat exactly the same amount of the same ingredients mixed with water. Scientists suspect this is because the water, while adding no calories, enhances flavors. The body (probably because of messages going to and from the hypothalamus) treats the tasty calories different. No one yet knows how this works.

Consuming artificial sweeteners with 0 calories can still lead to weight gain, because the taste of sweetness on our tongues causes our bodies to secrete more insulin so that we can digest the sugar the pancreas believes is on its way to our stomachs. All that insulin ends up rushing through our bloodstream like a jilted bride, searching desperately for the sugar that never shows up. We eat more food to balance the insulin, just as the bride might, understandably, sleep with an entire professional baseball team to compensate for her fiancé's desertion. (This was not the analogy used by the original researchers, but you take my point.)

RATS GAINED MORE ON BREAD THAN POWDER

Anyway, one consistent finding is that something called "sensory spe-cific satiety" makes us feel full. This is a fancy way of stating the well-known fact that when you eat a lot of food that has just one flavor, you get sick of that flavor. Your brain signals "enough, already!" and you feel stuffed. But toss in another flavor, and you'll come up with a little more appetite. This is why after a full meal of savory and salty food, a little something sweet can still be tasty.

Commercial food producers are well aware of this, so they pack foods with a variety of flavors to trick the brain into delaying that feeling of full-ness. That's why some chicken is infused with sugar water, while many cookies and cakes contain surprising amounts of salt; the more different tastes available from one food, the more of that food consumers will eat. My favorite study on sensory-specific satiety was done by NASA to determine which foods astronauts would still eat when zero gravity made them nause-ated. I won't bore you with the details; I'll just say that if you're planning a dinner party in outer space, serve Froot Loops, especially if all the guests are rats, and you plan to hang them by their tails before dinner is served. (In answer to the question that is no doubt arising in your mind: no, this test has not yet been replicated using lawyers.)

THE FLAVOR POINT DIET

Dr. David Katz, director of the Yale Prevention Research Center, has created a program called "the Flavor-Point Diet," the details of which are presented in a book of the same name. Dr. Katz offers many strategies for exploiting sensory-specific satiety, such as cutting out foods that have lots of complex flavor combinations and "draping" a single flavor over everything you eat on a specific day. On one day, you'll stick to foods that taste like cranberry; the next day is Lemon day, the next Pineapple day, etc. I tried this, and it really does cut your appetite. It's been spectacularly successful in helping its adherents lose weight. So if you want a terrific meal plan with lots of recipes, by all means try the Flavor Point Diet.

Sadly, I myself have far less cooking skill than your average vervet. I also have trouble with my hair-trigger famine brain when I limit each day's food to one basic flavor. What's more, I get bored. (I've found that boredom is one of the common reasons people go off the Atkins Diet. The food is so relentlessly meaty that the savory flavor receptors in the hypothalamus max out pretty quickly, resulting in sensory-specific satiety combined with a vague feeling that if you eat one more egg you will actually become a chicken.)

THE SHANGRI-LA DIET

Perhaps the weirdest advice that draws on flavor research is the "Shangri-la Diet," created by psychology professor Dr. Seth Roberts. Roberts believes that each person's body has a fat set point, which means that it "wants" to weigh a certain amount. There's persuasive research to support this theory: Overweight people who lose weight are likely to regain it, but when normal-weight people deliberately try to gain weight (for the sake of science), they actually have trouble doing so. Roberts believes that the set point of any given person can be manipulated by breaking the flavor-calorie association in the brain.

Here's the theory: Foods that are high in calories but have little or no flavor tell the body to *drop* your set point; foods with low calories and strong flavors *raise* your set point. This is ironic, because for decades diet books have been telling overweight people to satisfy their appetites by adding strong flavors to calorie-restricted diets—exactly the flavor strategy that (according to this theory) tells the body to put on more weight.

Roberts recommends that you do exactly the opposite: Fool your brain into lowering your set point by consuming small amounts of foods that have high calories but little to no flavor. Furthermore, he believes that pure sweetness doesn't count as a flavor. Here's his main diet strategy: After breakfast, go for at least 1 hour without putting any flavor in your mouth—no gum, no toothpaste, no iced tea, nothing. Then, consume either a tablespoon of flavorless olive oil or a tablespoon of sugar dissolved in several ounces of water. Then go at least 1 more hour without flavors. Other than that, you can eat whatever you want. You just (hypothetically) won't think about, crave, or consume as much food.

The reason I'm going into so much detail here is that when I experimented with it, the effect was amazing. I've never been less interested in food. Drinking oil or sugar water was disgusting, but I abruptly lost interest in all other rich or sugary foods. And me with my sweet tooth. So, though I truly didn't expect flavor manipulation to change my eating, I found it dramatically effective as an appetite suppressant. Now, many nutritionists think Dr. Roberts is so wrong that he should be imprisoned, preferably on death row. While good fats are actually very healthy, the suggestion about drink-ing sugar water makes steam spontaneously rise from the ears of dietitians.

So, if you want to try manipulating flavor to lose weight, I recommend an approach that's both easy and healthy. I call it flavor fasting. To diminish the physical sensation of hunger (this will have no effect on emotional eat-ing, which isn't appetite-based in the first place), first go at least 1 hour with no flavors—no toothpaste, no gum, no coffee, nothing. Then take some food supplements: two capsules of omega-3 fish oil, one of flaxseed oil, and one of vitamin E, which comes in oil form. It adds up to about ½ tablespoon of oil, all of it in forms that have been shown to be very, very good for us. Toss back all the supplements with 24 to 32 ounces of water. If you're thirsty, you might want to guzzle the water all at once, but for me, the appetite-suppressant effect works better if I sip the water over, say, a half-hour period. After you take the supplements, go at least another full hour without tasting any flavors.

The basis for my healthy eating is still psychological; if I don't constantly calm my mind and go to my Watcher self, I lose touch with my body's needs, and I may overeat. Since I'm not overweight at the moment, I don't restrict my eating at all and therefore don't often need flavor fasts. But on days when my weight's risen and I want to stop the trend, flavor fasting cuts my appe-tite considerably. Moreover, it seems to send me searching for interesting flavors. I end up eating—wanting—large amounts of stuff like blueberries and kale. I kid you not. Kale.

I had bloodwork done before and after an experimental period of flavor fasting. At the end of this period, my bad cholesterol and triglycerides were low, and my good cholesterol was high. All of this means I'm at lower risk of heart disease, though I may be killed by dietitians who discover I actually find Seth Roberts's suggestions useful. More research is needed to sort out the complex interaction effects of flavor, nutritional value, appetite, and body weight, but hang me by my tail and feed me Froot Loops, I think there's something to it.

EXERCISE: PLAY WITH FLAVOR

The preparation stage of your skinny lifestyle should include a little experi-mentation with flavor effects. You can buy the books written by Drs. Katz and/or Roberts, or you can just take their general advice by eating fewer complex flavor combinations. Both authors mention that delicately flavored foods tend to make us feel more satisfied more quickly than do foods with intense flavors. Food is less complexly flavored in its natural form than in prepared form, so choose food that isn't processed or mixed.

For example, if you would ordinarily eat a can of cake frosting each day at breakfast, try consuming the components separately: first a pound of sugar, then a stick of butter. No, no, I'm kidding! Don't eat any of those things! (Unless you are a vervet.) (Or a lawyer.) (Not really!)

Seriously, I highly recommend Dr. Katz's strategy of eating similarly flavored food during any given day. The recipes in *The Flavor Point Diet* will serve you well if this strategy appeals, so stock up on the foods you'll need to make those dishes. If you want to join me in my flavor fasting, please ask your doctor about it and experiment carefully to see how it affects your health indicators, as well as your appetite and food choices.

Along with formal observation techniques like blood tests, direct the close attention of the Watcher toward your own body. Notice how you feel after eating foods with various flavors. Observe how you pig out on sugary food when you're already stuffed with salty stuff or eat six bowls of cold cereal at one sitting. Pay attention to the emotions that go along with the consumption of different flavors. Above all, remember to offer kindness to the parts of you that lust after certain foods and avoid others. Stay in Watcher mode. Keep breathing, and observe any anxiety that arises until it crests and recedes. You'll need your self-calming skills at the ready as we move into the next chapter.

"Flavor Fast" 4-Day Win

Ridiculously Easy Daily Goal: _Each day for the next 4 days, I'll experiment_

with flavor. I'll either (1) eat similarly flavored foods all day long; (2) have a 2

hour flavor fast with a dose of water, healthy supplements, and fiber; or (3) both

of the above. I'll pay close attention to the way my body reacts to flavors, knowing

this will strongly impact my eventual attempts to eat less.

Small Daily Reward: _____

_____

Slightly Larger 4-Day Reward: _____

_____

	Dates of My Current 4-Day Win	**Check Off Completed Days Here**
Day 1:	____ / ____ / ____	_____
Day 2:	____ / ____ / ____	_____
Day 3:	____ / ____ / ____	_____
Day 4:	____ / ____ / ____	_____

   If you're already on a weight-loss regimen, remember that the 4-day win will enhance it, not conflict with it. If you know what to do, this program will help you do what you know. Feel free to stay on any weight-loss program while you learn 4-day win skills!

CHAPTER 25

WHAT'S MY MOTIVATION?

MAKING MOVING EASIER

I'm writing these words at the gym, in a notebook, during the 47-second break between sets of crunches. I love the gym. No phones or e-mails interrupt me, and there's a blessed simplicity to pedaling a stationary bike or heaving pieces of metal. What I do not like at the gym is company. I never take a workout buddy. I never go to an exercise class. The only thing a personal trainer might motivate me to do is run away. I am an exercise loner, and the few occasions when I've tried working out with other people have made me grumpy. For me, solitude is a huge motivator.

My friend Delia has a very different exercise-motivation profile. A college athlete who'd stopped exercising when she had kids, Delia spent years telling her husband, Sam, "I should go to the gym." Finally, he bought her a membership for several hundred dollars. Even with this added guilt, she rarely managed to show up for a workout, and when she did, her efforts were half-baked and ineffective. Sam, undaunted, bought her a set of three appointments with a personal trainer. Delia loved every minute of these sessions. When Sam suggested hiring the trainer permanently, Delia protested that this would be self-indulgent and too expensive. "I'll tell you what would be expensive," said Sam. "All the medical care you'll need if you never exercise." Delia hired the trainer, and she's hardly missed a workout in 5 years.

Exercise is effort, and effort, as any actor will tell you, makes no sense unless it's seriously motivated. But different people are motivated by different things. There are two personality factors that, in my observation, combine to determine the type of motivation people need to begin and sustain a

207

higher level of physical activity. The first is "conative style," a way of taking action that differs between individuals. The second is social interaction style—how you like to connect with other people. We're going to use these two variables to figure out your motivation style, preparing you to move more for the rest of your natural life.

EXPLANATION: CONATION AND ASSOCIATION

Aristotle and a host of his intellectual successors divided human consciousness into three components: the affective (feeling), the cognitive (thinking), and the "conative," which addresses the manner of action (doing). The world's most accomplished conative theorist, Kathy Kolbe, has done decades of research that indicates that human action styles break down into characteristic types. Understanding how conative styles work is helpful in any number of arenas, so I enthusiastically suggest you visit Kathy Kolbe's Web site (www.kolbe.com) or read her books to learn much more than I can tell you here.

The reason I bring up this issue is that knowing your conative style facilitates your preparation for moving more—specifically, your choice of an exercise program. Below you'll find a very rough description of the—surprise!—four basic conative patterns. All humans are capable of operating in all ways, but most of us favor one or two conative patterns and are less comfortable with others. You can take an online test at Kathy Kolbe's Web site to get a detailed analysis of your conative style, but for now, read through the following typologies and see which type sounds most like you.

CONATIVE TYPES (KOLBE'S CATEGORIES)

- *Fact Finder:* When Fact Finders set out to start an activity—in this case, exercising more—they start by looking for *information*. They do research, study, ask lots and lots of questions, and don't feel comfortable moving on without total understanding of what they're attempting.
- *Follow Thru:* A person who favors Follow Thru conative behavior is most comfortable working with *systems*. Follow Thru's are the people

who set up libraries, educational systems, military procedures. They like rules and order, which they follow almost perfectly. They dislike chaotic, improvised, or unstructured action.

- *Quick Start:* Quick Starts work with pure *action.* They jump right in and get started, even without full information or structure, figuring they'll learn by trial and error. They tend to be creative, since they don't necessarily follow the rules or wait for precedent to be established.

- *Implementers:* Implementers work through concrete *objects.* They build models of DNA or satellites, put their bodies in motion, and are excellent at things that require physical participation. Abstraction is less interesting to them than concrete reality.

As I've mentioned, all of us can do all these behaviors in a pinch, but you probably favor one or two conative approaches and may have one you actively dislike. I, for example, am predominantly a Quick Start. I'm comfortable in a Fact Finder or Implementer mode, but I strongly resist systematic Follow Thru behavior. (If you're a Follow Thru or a Fact Finder, you probably won't even want to choose your own conative style without more information or structure, so by all means, visit Kathy Kolbe's Web site.) If you play to your innate type when choosing an exercise program, you'll be more likely to get moving. Here's some advice:

- *Fact Finder:* If you're a Fact Finder, go ahead and find facts. You've probably read a lot of books like this one, and you spend lots of time online, ferreting out all kinds of information on anything that interests you. If you're a sociable sort, quiz experts: trainers, doctors, physical therapists, athletes, trusted friends. Keep gathering information until you're satisfied that you have a working knowledge of an exercise program that will fit snugly into your life.

  Do . . . keep asking questions until you start hearing the same information repeated over and over. That means you've begun to master your topic, and you'll make a good choice.

  Don't . . . get stuck in what Kathy Kolbe calls "analysis paralysis," thinking you'll act after you get just a little more information . . . and a little more . . . and a little more. . . . Get a Quick Start friend or trainer to push you into action if you aren't moving on your own (see your social style on the following pages to help choose the right person).

- *Follow Thru:* You probably won't consistently move more until you're plugged into a system, preferably where you spend money or make promises to a trainer or teammates. Sign up for a class (dance, yoga, sports, clown school, anything that interests you) or hire a professional instructor who takes a very structured approach.

  Do . . . set goals: Train for a race or competition, climb a mountain. Or try tackling a new skill you've always wanted to learn. If you're an experienced exerciser already, consider becoming a trainer, yoga teacher, or diving instructor. Whatever your abilities, take them to the next level.

  Don't . . . try to improvise a workout program without strong goals or some kind of structured program. You thrive in a boot camp environment; getting all loosey-goosey just won't motivate you effectively.

- *Quick Start:* Follow Nike's advice: Just Do It. If anything sounds interesting to you—if you find yourself feeling tugged toward rowing or ice skating or the flying trapeze—get some basic instructions, then set aside some time and make up a workout as you go along. Just be sure that you never take physical risks without instruction, supervision, and whatever sort of safety harness, boots, helmet, aqualung, or suit of armor is recommended.

  Do . . . hang loose, have lots of fun, and constantly modify your program based on what is and isn't working for you. Try lots of different activities until you find one that keeps you right on the edge of being too challenged. Switch activities if you get bored.

  Don't . . . think you should follow a set of rules that makes you feel hemmed in. Classes and instructors that work well for your Follow Thru friends might be demotivating for you. If you exercise with others, make sure they're at least as wild as you are.

- *Implementers:* If you like gadgets, gizmos, and special sports clothing, you're strong in Implementer skills, and you should exploit them to get yourself moving. Choose a workout activity that requires neat stuff—a bicycle, a five-dollar pedometer, a pair of skates, a horse, a set of numchucks, and a sword. Don't let yourself play with these things unless you're engaging in your "move more" workout program—and you've had adequate instruction and supervision.

     Do . . . learn to use lots of different activity-related objects, even if you have to rent rather than own. Spend plenty of time checking out the newest model of stretch-resistance bands or stopwatches or hiking gear. Use gizmos as rewards for 4-day wins.

     Don't . . . force yourself to do activities that require lots of mental calculations, like adding up the calories burned at various paces and distances or keeping batting averages in your head. As an Implementer, you're already a very physically grounded person, and almost any physical action is likely to be fairly motivating to you—as long as you respect personal fascinations and one other factor: social style.

SOCIAL STYLES

The "affective" part of consciousness has a strong influence on how we interact with other people. The folks you hang with when you're moving are the strongest external force in sustaining a frisky lifestyle. I've noticed four (what is it with that number?) distinct social patterns that my clients prefer when it comes to exercise:

- *Lone Rangers:* You're a Lone Ranger if, like me, you prefer to exercise alone. Lone Rangers are actually thrilled by solitude during exercise; company or supervision bothers them. In sports, they're the distance runners, swimmers, solo rock climbers.

     Exercise Motivators: If you're a Lone Ranger, you'll be most motivated by carving out selfish space in your schedule for exercise. Even if you feel a bit guilty, make your workout time—even if it's just D-level fidgeting—all yours. No interruptions, no company. Try listening to music or audiobooks when (and only when) you're exercising.

- *Partner People:* Some people love to exercise with just one other person: a training partner, spouse, spotter, trainer, coach. If you're a partner person, you may also like playing games, like racquet sports or pickup basketball, that pit you against one other person. Or you may prefer the more lyrical movement of dance or partner yoga.

    Exercise Motivators: Make a commitment to one other person that you'll show up to exercise with him/her. If your spouse, sibling or best buddy is up for the challenge, that's fine. But it's actually more motivating to make a promise to a person you don't know as well, particularly someone you're paying. The more formal the relationship, the less likely you'll beg out of it. Think like Sam: Paying money to a trainer now is better than paying more money to a doctor later in your life.

- *Team Players:* Team players are the archetypal jocks; they love the "band of brothers/sisters" feeling of team sports. They'll join pickup games with strangers rather than exercise alone. They're motivated by any situation where a group of folks is exercising together with a common goal.

    Exercise Motivators: Obviously, you need a team. If you're not a pro athlete, you can find or establish an informal team for your favorite sport or for line dancing, cheerleading, cow tipping, etc. Oprah's famous "spa girls" met daily to exercise for over a year, targeting group goals like running a half-marathon (you can find details about how to set up your own "spa girls" group on www.oprah.com).

- *Crowd Pleasers:* These are people who both please crowds and are pleased by them. Their idea of a good time is a rowdy club. They get motivated by things like a "Slim Down This Town!" initiative, a media challenge (*Body for Life, The Biggest Loser*), or the latest exercise craze.

Exercise Motivators: Go where the fun is—road races, dance clubs, classes in aerobics, jazzercize, kick-boxing, Tae Bo. Crowd pleasers also do well in semi-structured environments like the Curves circuit-training gyms, where women congregate informally to do resistance training under the supervision of helpful trainers.

So, have you identified a favorite association style? As with your conative patterns, you may be capable of enjoying all kinds of workouts, but you'll gravitate most toward one or two. Choose the conative and associative patterns that you think best describe you. Keep both in mind as you do your next 4-day win, which is making specific plans for increasing your activity level—and staying motivated for the long term.

EXERCISE: MOTION MOTIVATION

There are—yes, indeedy—four components you need to get fully prepared for a new exercise program: a structured program, good advice and information, a place in which to move, and equipment (if only loose clothes and a floor). As you may have noticed, these correspond to the conative styles. Depending on what interests you, movement-wise, you may have more of one element than another. For example, if you decide to take regular walks, your primary need will be location, though shoes (equipment), time (structure), and information (how long should you walk per day and how fast?) will also play a role. If you decide to go skydiving, you better damn well have the right equipment, a very structured learning program, and excellent information. As for location, well . . . the sky. Not much to decide there. At any rate, you should begin creating a plan to move more by playing to your conative strength. If your type is . . .

- *Implementer:* Start with equipment. Go to a sporting goods store, a yoga studio's clothing shop, a music store where you can buy your favorite dance music. Talk to the people who sell or use these things, and let them direct you to the systems, information sources, and locations where your move-more escapades can begin.

- *Quick Start:* Begin by going to the location where an activity takes place; a studio, a hiking trail, a ski resort. There you'll find experts, systems, and equipment that will get you started on your activity.
- *Fact Finder:* Begin by accessing the most authoritative information source available in cyberspace, in print, or in real life. Find yourself an expert—or a few experts—who can tell you where to go for your chosen activity, what equipment you'll need, and how to tap into a structured program that will give you some milestones and goals.
- *Follow Thru:* Find a system such as a class, a trainer, or a structured workout program that you can connect with. Join a walking club in your neighborhood. Enter a get-in-shape competition. Hire support in the form of trainers, teachers, physical therapists, anyone who can help you increase your mobility with a sense of support.

So your 4-day win for this phase of preparation is to spend 30 minutes each day creating a move-more plan. You'll start by accessing whatever loop you need to get set up in the way that's dictated by your conative style. Within your chosen activity (or activities), create social space—solitude, partnership, teamwork, or a whole crowd—that makes you feel most excited about this new level of physical action. Remember, you're not just doing some nasty exercise to drop some weight so that you can go back to normal life. This increased level of physical activity is your new normal. And you can prepare to move by setting up a situation where that's much more exciting than the normal you've had until now.

"Motion Motivation" 4-Day Win

Ridiculously Easy Daily Goal: *Each day for the next 4 days, I'll spend half an hour preparing the details of my move-more initiative, starting from my conative strength and connecting with people or groups who are most motivating to me. By Day 4, I'll have a plan that feels highly motivating.*

Small Daily Reward: _____

_____

Slightly Larger 4-Day Reward: _____

_____

	Dates of My Current 4-Day Win	**Check Off Completed Days Here**
Day 1:	__ / __ / __	_____
Day 2:	__ / __ / __	_____
Day 3:	__ / __ / __	_____
Day 4:	__ / __ / __	_____

If you're already on a weight-loss regimen, remember that the 4-day win will enhance it, not conflict with it. If you know what to do, this program will help you do what you know. Feel free to stay on any weight-loss program while you learn 4-day win skills!

CHAPTER 26

YOU'RE GETTING VERRRRY SLEEEEPYYY . . .

AVOIDING BURNOUT

Z oe was a high-powered investment banker who came to one of my seminars to shake off the despondency she'd developed after years of unsuccessful fertility treatments. Though both Zoe and her husband had checked out as medically capable breeders, they'd been trying to get pregnant for years without success. They'd spent a fortune on everything from hormone injections to in vitro fertilizations, but all Zoe's poked, prodded, and forcibly impregnated body had managed to produce was one conception that ended in a miscarriage.

Zoe was a tough cookie, and in the midst of all this pain and heartbreak, she'd miraculously come up with the energy to be great at her job. By the time I met her, she was a very high-ranking, wealthy woman. She was also a bit chubby. She'd gained over 40 pounds between the ages of 30 and 35. She'd hired a personal trainer and trained for a marathon, but though she finished the race 6 months later, she'd actually gained another pound.

I was more interested in Zoe's quality of life than her weight. She chatted with energetic charm, but you got the feeling it was an act, and a fragile one at that. By late afternoon, she was so obviously running on fumes that I just up and asked her about it. Zoe crumpled like a deflated paper bag. It all came out: the infertility trauma, the depression, the weight gain. The next question seemed obvious to everyone in the room except Zoe.

"Are you sleeping enough?" I asked.

"Enough?" Zoe's brow furrowed. "I guess so. Whatever 'enough' means."

"'Enough' means that you sleep until you're not tired anymore," I explained.

Zoe chuckled drily. "Are you kidding? I've been tired since I was about 12."

"So how many hours do you sleep every night?"

"I don't sleep every night," she said. "But on the nights I go to bed, I'd say I get between 2 and 5 hours."

Everyone in the room gasped.

"What?" said Zoe, looking at our horrified expressions. "Listen, you guys don't get what it's like in my business. I swim with sharks. Plus, I've taken a lot of time off for the medical stuff. And I have to get up at 5 every morning to run. I mean, I'm gaining weight as it is. If I didn't work out, I'd really be a whale."

Zoe was brilliant but also grievously misinformed. She really thought that health and slenderness came from dietary deprivation and constant maximum performance in personal and professional life. A lot of smart people believe this, particularly Americans. I think it goes back to the Protestant ethic, which sociologist Max Weber saw as the dominant cultural model of the United States. Minimize pleasure, maximize work; that's the Protestant ethic in a nutshell. Most of us follow it until it's just too frigging much trouble—approximately 15 minutes—then lie down and eat bonbons to keep up our strength. But some people go too far the other way.

Here's a plain fact that rarely comes up in American treatises on weight loss: Dieting and exercising too much can cause weight gain, as well as a host of degenerative illnesses. In fact, it may be just as damaging to be too active and abstemious as it is to lounge around like a slug. Many people, driven by intensely competitive, high-achieving cultural norms, discipline themselves into being fat, immobile, depressed, and sometimes very sick. You may think of it simply as inordinate exhaustion. But its more specific name is "adrenal burnout," and learning to recognize and fend it off is an essential part of your preparation for losing weight.

EXPLANATION: THE PERILS OF BEING POOPED

The fight-or-flight response comes from complex hormonal changes that occur almost instantly when we realize we're in danger. But the same things happen when we get very excited in a positive way, say by dancing all night at a crowded club or working in a very intense, high-pressure environment. When you're in any extremely stimulating situation, your neocortex sends the message "Wow! Look what's happening!" to the limbic system, which produces an emotion such as fear: "Oh, God, I'm gonna die!" or ecstasy: "I am the dancing queen! Feel the beat! Of the tambourine! Oh, yeah!"

At this point your hypothalamus sends a message to your autonomic nervous system, which causes your adrenal glands to pump a whole lot of adrenaline (epinephrine and norepinephrine) into your blood. You also produce stress hormones like cortisol and glucocorticoids. Your whole body reacts: Your heart rate and blood pressure go up, you tremble, your throat goes dry, your palms sweat. All of these responses evolved to help you survive in extreme emergencies. (Interesting point: Sweaty palms, which make your grip weaker on artificial surfaces like smooth plastic or metal, increase your gripping capacity on natural surfaces like rocks and branches.) Your adrenal glands can't produce an infinite supply of pick-me-up hormones; if you're burning through them all the time, you eventually get only a trickle, not a flood. You've now reached adrenal burnout.

Pushing ourselves to extremes can keep us in a near-permanent state of fight-or-flight response. This level of exhaustion is like being run over by a steamroller very, very slowly. At first you hardly notice it—you're just a little tired and cranky. Then you can't get up without coffee every day. Then the coffee stops helping, even when you add several candy bars. Then you get eye bags the size and color of mature eggplants. Then you start crying whenever you have to get out of bed. Then you develop muscle tearing, viral infections, memory loss, and an inability to read anything longer than haiku. Then you fall over in the Phoenix airport and have to be taken to the hospital, where they install you in the emergency room next to a man with nine fingers who's being interrogated by the police with questions that include: "So what happened after the second time he shot you?" At least, this is the way I personally experienced it (really) during my most recent burnout experience.

I've seen this happen to other authors on book tours, to singers who create adrenaline rushes for crowds every night, to politicians, pro athletes, TV producers. I think it's the reason stimulant abuse is so common in these professions. And then there's the most pressured job in the world: caring for small children, especially without other adults around. I've worked with suburban soccer moms who began smoking crack (again, I'm serious) to perform "perfectly" in their roles.

Here's the thing: If you religiously followed many diet-and-exercise programs found in the more aggressive fitness magazines, you'd put yourself directly in the path of adrenal burnout. Professional athletes burn out this way unless they take time off, then train to a peak for specific events. Trying to peak all the time lands you in the valley, yea, verily, the valley of the shadow of death.

As you get closer to total adrenal burnout, your body tries, with increasing desperation, to make you rest and recuperate. You feel fatigued, then exhausted. Without arousal hormones left for normal use, you're also dejected and joyless. Your elevated cortisol levels break down muscle tissue, and because you're under constant pressure, your body can't produce enough healing hormones (like DHEA) to repair this breakdown. You get mouth sores. Small cuts don't heal. Muscle strength deteriorates, and you may injure yourself. Incongruously, you develop insomnia. Your metabolism slows, and calories that were once burned up are now stored as fat. *The very things that once made you healthier, stronger, and fitter are now making you unhealthier, weaker, and fatter.* If you persist in overstressing without rest, your immune system will falter or even turn against you, making you vulnerable to all sorts of illness, from colds to cancer.

Zoe confirmed that in addition to depression and weight gain, she'd also experienced a lot of viral infections, constant canker sores, and a series of running injuries. Here's what really blew me away: Zoe told me that throughout all those zillion-dollar fertility treatments, no medical personnel had asked if she had burnout symptoms or even if she got enough sleep. Maybe Zoe just didn't remember correctly, but she might have been right. Possibly, her doctors were so focused on looking at things like ovulation that they weren't using evolutionary logic (why would any female body take on the incredibly taxing job of having a baby when there's too little food and too much exercise, which indicates some sort of emergency?). Then there's the fact that *American doctors aren't trained to see being tired and wired as a problem.* They're forced to undergo high-pressure situations with inadequate sleep from medical school all the way through residency—and to consider triumphing over exhaustion virtuous. Even more than the rest of us, they're actually trained to see burnout as a virtue.

If you live on the edge of exhaustion, have an intense job, work out regularly, eat sparingly, and are putting on weight while feeling progressively crappier, you're courting adrenal burnout. If you're so tired, weak, injured, and depressed you can hardly move, you and burnout have gone past the courting stage, taken vows, and moved in together. You have married an axe murderer. It's time to get divorced. Depending on how burnt out you are, you may have to temporarily move *less* and eat *more* of certain foods in order to lose weight.

Our cultural bias against this is so strong that I have a hell of a time convincing my clients to try it. Zoe fought hard against my suspicion that she was adrenally burnt out, but eventually she started believing me. And then she did something fabulous: She fell asleep, sitting up, right there in the seminar. The next day she bought an excellent book that I assign as mandatory reading for all clients with symptoms of burnout: *Tired of Being Tired,* by Jesse Lynn Hadley, MD. *If any of the discussion above rings a bell for you, buy this book today.* You'll find an excellent, detailed version of the information I'll run through briefly below.

EXERCISE: CHECKING FOR BURNOUT

Dr. Hanley offers a diagnostic quiz to check for adrenal-burnout symptoms, as well as a rating system to see how burnt out you are and suggestions for recovery at every level. See if any of Hanley's "five stages of burnout" describe you.

Dr. Hanley's Five-Level Burnout Description

Driven: You're a high achiever and stress junky, doing difficult things and doing them well. You either exercise like a maniac, or you're so busy with other things, you don't get much exercise at all. You eat a lot of junk food because it's easy to grab on the fly. You've started using caffeine and/or smoking to stay sharp, but you look and feel great.

Dragging: You're feeling a little worn around the edges, a bit tired and achy-breaky. You drink caffeine first thing every morning to get going. You sometimes eat junk as a pick-me-up, as well as for meals. If you smoke, you're going through more cigarettes. Even if you exercise, you're feeling a little flabby. Sometimes, when you really have to perform, you swig a high-caffeine sports drink or even use some form of stimulant, from ephedra to cocaine.

Losing It: You have dark circles under your eyes, you're gaining weight even though you're dieting, and you can't sleep well. Your usual high-octane, fun personality has become darker; you brood, worry, and sometimes feel intense anxiety that makes your heart race. You get angry or weepy when pushed too far. No amount of caffeine or other form of uppers helps much.

Hitting the Wall: You have come to resemble Uncle Fester on *The Addams Family*. You whine nonstop—to yourself or others—about how tired you are, how fat you've gotten, and how meaningless and terrifying your life feels. You can't remember anything. Exercise is rare and feels awful. You're having stomach trouble, joint trouble, headache trouble, and relationship trouble. People walk on eggshells to keep from setting off your anxiety or anger, and then you get anxious and angry because you hate people walking on eggshells. Nobody likes you.

Burned Out: You've fallen, and you can't get up. All you want to do is lie in bed and cry. You're sick all the time—with minor illnesses if you're lucky, major ones, like heart disease or cancer, if you're not. You may have developed an autoimmune disorder, irritable bowel syndrome, fibromyalgia, interstitial cystitis, arthritis, or other crippling conditions. You feel you have nothing to live for anyway. You're horribly lonely, because along with puffiness and premature aging, you display all the happy-go-lucky interpersonal warmth of a piranha.

If any of the descriptions above describes you, it is imperative that you address adrenal burnout before you start any program of eating less and moving more. For example, if you're at full burnout, exercise will make things worse; what you need most is sleep. Lots of it. Ten hours a night, plus daytime naps. Talk to a doctor who knows about adrenal burnout, read anything you can find on the topic, including Dr. Hanley's book, and take the suggestions you find there. Until you restore your adrenal system, nothing in all of the diet-and-exercise literature will work for you. You'll gain weight while eating less and exercising more, if only because you're creating so much tissue inflammation that you retain large amounts of fluid.

Though the full response necessary to heal adrenal burnout is beyond this book's scope, I use a trick called "minimum days" to help at any stage. Give it a try for 4 days. If you've been experiencing burnout, you'll feel better physically and emotionally, and oddly enough (considering that you'll be eating more and moving less), your weight gain will stop or reverse itself.

MINIMUM DAYS

Take a weekend or call in sick for a couple of days, or (best of all) take 2 sick days right next to a weekend. During those 4 days, do only the absolute minimum work required to keep yourself alive and—if you can't get a sitter—care for kids or pets. I mean *minimum*. No getting dressed. No laundry, housecleaning, catching up on correspondence, doing favors for friends. *Nada!* If you feel anxious or compulsive about getting things done even though you feel like carrion, become the Watcher. Get peaceful. Watch yourself. Note the panic you feel about being active, your fear of simply being, without distraction. Consider chatting about this with a therapist. Stay in the identity of the compassionate Watcher until the "get something done!" panic abates. It probably won't last longer than 15 minutes.

The only thing you're allowed to do on a minimum day, other than creep to the potty every so often, is to lie in bed, watching mindless TV or reading something totally unimpressive, and nibble on healthy food all day long. Don't limit your calories, carbs, or fat grams; just eat a little healthy food whenever you feel peckish. Here's how to tell if minimum days are working:

By the end of Day 1: You feel the stirring of hope.

By the end of Day 2: You're crying less, and you keep falling into restful sleep.

By the end of Day 3: You remember wanting to do things. You can smile.

By the end of Day 4: You want to live. Also, you weigh less.

Mind you, I'm not suggesting minimum days for someone who's never been active. This strategy is for people who show signs of constant acceleration, emotional and physical revving, accompanied by inexplicable inability to stop gaining weight. The acid test is that, even though you may eat more than you're used to during minimum days and you'll hardly move at all, your weight will have dropped by Day 4.

Minimum days are a backfield skill I need every time my weight creeps up in concert with high levels of stress and effort. They may be enough for you, or you may need to do a full-on recovery from adrenal burnout before your weight issues stop being all bass-ackwards. That's what Zoe did. Ever the high performer, she found out all about adrenal burnout and put her intense drive into caring for herself as well as she would care for a child. Which is a very good thing, because I understand her new baby is really cute.

"Minimum Movement" 4-Day Win

(For Folks with Burnout Symptoms Only)

Ridiculously Easy Daily Goal: *Each day for the next 4 days, I'll cancel all nonessential activities, lie in bed wearing my jammies, enjoy mindless entertainment, nibble on healthy food whenever I feel hungry. If I feel anxious and want to get up, I'll go to the place of Thinner Peace until the feeling passes.*

Small Daily Reward: _____

_____

Slightly Larger 4-Day Reward: _____

_____

	Dates of My Current 4-Day Win	Check Off Completed Days Here
Day 1:	___ / ___ / ___	_____
Day 2:	___ / ___ / ___	_____
Day 3:	___ / ___ / ___	_____
Day 4:	___ / ___ / ___	_____

If you're already on a weight-loss regimen, remember that the 4-day win will enhance it, not conflict with it. If you know what to do, this program will help you do what you know. Feel free to stay on any weight-loss program while you learn 4-day win skills!

CHAPTER 27

YOU NEED
NEW MOVES

PREPARING TO MOVE MORE

Exhibit One: Caroline. She sits down across from me at Starbucks look-ing zippy as a red convertible in her new Nike outfit. "I feel so much better since I started exercising!" she says.

"That's great!" I say. "What kind of workout are you doing?"

"Well, I run for an hour on the treadmill, then I head over to the coun-try club and take a spin class and a Pilates class. After that I hit the gym for some weight training, and I'm done for the day!" she sips a green tea that's bursting with antioxidants. "I should lose 3 pounds a week if I stick to the program."

"Wait a second," I say. "You just started exercising, and you're doing 4 hours a day?"

"Absolutely!" Caroline beams.

Two weeks later, I see her again. She's wearing another adorable workout suit. Other than that, she looks like a cautionary illustration in a pamphlet on chronic fatigue syndrome. Her eyes are half-shut, her posture slumped, her expression pained.

"I don't know what's wrong with me," she groans, tossing back a venti quadruple-shot espresso. "My get-up-and-go just got up and went." She orders another coffee. "And you know what really pisses me off, Martha? I weighed myself this morning, and I've only lost a pound! This makes no sense! I work out 4 hours a day for this? I'm furious!"

"Dude," I said, "you're overtraining."

"Ridiculous," she says. "I've got to lose weight. To lose weight, you work out. Period!"

Later that day, Caroline develops a severe back spasm and has to stop exercising entirely.

Exhibit Two: my son Adam. Like many teens with Down syndrome, Adam's genetically low muscle tone predisposes him to weight gain. But Adam looks pretty damn fit due to his participation in Special Olympics and predilection for hip-hop.

"Mom," Adam says when I get home from having coffee with Caroline, "I need this." He gives me a piece of paper on which he has painstakingly copied an 800 number. I look at the number, knowing that if I call it, I'll end up spending money. God knows what commercial has convinced Adam he needs something new—a George Foreman grill, an adjustable bed, breast implants. "Did you see this on TV?" I ask.

He nods.

"Well, what do you want me to buy for you?"

"Dance video," he says.

"But you already have a lot of dance videos."

"Not that one."

"Are you really sure you'll use it?"

Adam looks at me with the beginning of alarm in his eyes. Then he says in a voice quivering with fervor, "Mom! I need new moves!"

Now it's 6 months later, and you should see that boy dance.

EXPLANATION: ENDOGENOUS EXERCISE

The difference between Caroline and Adam is the difference between a person who exercises in spurts, never making exercise a habitual part of a long-term lifestyle, and someone who's likely to stay physically active forever. Caroline's whole approach to moving more is based on media stereotypes of athleticism. She imagines herself looking and exercising like the fitness models in magazines and TV—*right now*. Her model of "an athletic person" is exogenous (coming from outside her experience) and makes her exercise too much or not at all.

Adam's exercise program, by contrast, is endogenous. It consists of activities—not always athletic—that he's always loved. Adam dances almost every day, sometimes with friends, sometimes alone with his Wal-Mart karaoke machine. He participates in the Special Olympics events—bowling, basketball, and especially swimming—that are fun for him. He sometimes pushes himself to exhaustion, but only for competitive events. Case in point: As I was writing this, Adam walked past on his way to swim practice.

"Are you going to work out hard?" I asked him.

Adam replied, "Not very hard. I'd get sick. Then I couldn't win medals."

And he, not Caroline, is supposed to be "intellectually challenged."

GREAT EXPECTATIONS, LOUSY RESULTS

As a culture, we share more of Caroline's exercise psychology than Adam's. We want to look and move like top athletes on cover shots. We forget that many of those gorgeous bodies owe their chiseled perfection to photographic retouching, steroids, or eating disorders. We ignore the fact that the careers of high-intensity athletes are usually short and painful. Remember O. J. Simpson's legal defense team claiming he couldn't have killed Nicole because he was too crippled to do anything more upsetting than a vague scowl? Most football players, as well as other pro athletes, train with an intensity that leaves them seriously damaged. Even track greyhounds and racehorses often exit, limping, after a brief candle of a career.

When you get to the action stage of your 4-day win program, you'll move more—but along Adam's lines, not Caroline's. Building your most effective personal exercise program may involve thousand-dollar outfits and hours of training a day, but *it will work*. You'll just do a bit more of something you already enjoy, repeat for 4 days, then increase by another small increment. In theory, this may seem frustratingly slow to you. It did to Caroline, which is why she's been sidelined with back trouble for months now. That, I promise you, is where real frustration sets in. If you're willing to be more tortoise than hare, you'll be fit enough for intense workouts sooner, and you'll stay fit longer. Forever.

FOUR KINDS OF 4-DAY WORKOUTS

I have several diagnosed conditions that are all poorly understood, but thought to be autoimmune diseases. The most debilitating of these is pervasive, excruciating pain in my soft tissues, which has fewer visible symptoms than some of my other symptoms (interstitial cystitis, granuloma annulari) but has seriously interfered with my well-laid plans for physical fitness. My doctors call it fibromyalgia. I call it other names, none of which

I can write down in a family book. An attack of this condition feels like a really, really bad sore throat—the kind that makes it agonizing to swallow—in various large sections of my body.

Because of this condition, there have been many years when I couldn't walk, couldn't lift things, couldn't so much as bend over without almost blacking out from pain. So I tend to feel frustrated by fitness books and magazines—frustrated for myself and for all the other people out there who have some sort of disease or disability that keeps us from dashing around like navy SEALS, whether or not we want to. I spent most of my twenties lying in bed, twitching and panting to distract myself from pain, longing for the days when I ran a minimum of 7 miles a day. I would have given every dollar I owned for the ability to follow the instructions I saw in fitness magazines. But the reality for most of us is that there will be times when our bodies just can't take the stress of serious workouts.

That's why I'd like you to have different workout programs in mind, each customized to fit your particular exercise preferences. Workout A will be like Caroline's ideal: a major aerobic and strength-training program, complete with gear, special locations, support people, and high intensity. Workout B is the kind of exercise a good trainer would advise you to do on a day you were busy or tired. Workout C is what you'll do when you can't fit in any kind of formal exercise session or when you're feeling out of sorts. Workout D is reserved for bad days, when you're so busy with work or family you barely have time to breathe or when you're so tired that it's an effort just to get up off the couch. The option below Workout D is a minimum day.

When it's time for you to go into action (in a couple of chapters), I'd like you to start doing the workout one stage *easier* than what you think is doable. *When beginning to move more (or to eat less), an easy 4-day win, followed by a slightly harder 4-day win, etc., is the key to genuinely improving your overall condition.* If you only do D workouts every day for the rest of your life, you'll be thinner than if you jump straight to A workouts before your body is ready. I started with D workouts—sometimes just lying down and doing a few passive stretches—and found that 4-day wins resulted in a very, very gradual training effect that made my body stronger without pitching me into pain or injury. After years of 4-day wins, all very gradual, I can actually do a lot of the routines in fitness magazines. But when I'm tired, I either drop down to a lower-effort workout or pay the consequences, by which I mean flare-ups of pain that feel like a deranged homeopath is trying to perform acupuncture on my entire body using railroad spikes.

So now, let's specify what constitutes A, B, C, and D workouts for you. We're going to work backward, from the easiest move-more option to the most strenuous.

EXERCISE: CREATING YOUR MOVE-MORE OPTIONS

WORKOUT D: AUGMENTED FIDGETING

Consider this: If you ran 3.5 miles today, you'd burn about 350 calories. If you're an average jogger, this would take about half an hour of dedicated time (meaning you couldn't do much else simultaneously) and require good shoes, tolerable weather, decent terrain, or a treadmill. It would take quite a toll on your muscles and joints. You'd probably want to change clothes and shower.

Or, you could just fidget.

That was the finding of a 2005 study at the Mayo Clinic. People who engage in commonplace mundane bodily movements, such as standing up to stretch, pacing while waiting for a call to go through, or throwing harpoons at their office managers, burn 350 more calories a day than people who sit still. That's the equivalent of losing up to 30 pounds a year, just by breaking the rules we all learned in kindergarten.

So, I'd like to propose that your D workout consist of escalated fidgeting within the course of a normal day. The tendency to fidget is partly inborn, but the Mayo researchers point out that anyone can increase fidgeting from a personal baseline just as we were all forced to *decrease* from our baselines as kids. To recall your favorite fidgeting techniques, you may have to go back to your preschool days. But your skills are still there, quashed though they might have been by decades of schooling and socially appropriate (read: fattening) behavior.

I myself am prone to pacing, jiggling one foot, absentmindedly petting dogs, and drawing or painting pictures (which doesn't sound fidgety until you realize that I'm constantly backing away from my pictures to see how they look from a distance, then rushing forward to fix the problems I've spotted, then backing off again). I don't do these things all the time, but when I do fidget, they are my preferred forms. My friend Betsy specializes in what she calls "deliberate inefficiency," making several unnecessary trips up and down the stairs instead of making a single well-planned journey with laundry, mail, schoolbooks, things to file, etc. What about you?

FAVORITE FIDGETS

Please write down at least three ways in which you like to fidget. Behaviors that first appeared in childhood are especially useful. List as many as you can:

_____

_____

_____

_____

WORKOUT C: STROLLING ABOUT

The residents of New York City are leaner than the average non–Big Apple American, partly because they walk more. The rest of the United States? One big car town. So although taking a nice walk outside is an ideal C-level workout, you may live in a place where that's not realistic. Or you may hate walking just for walking's sake. So walk for a reason. Our primordial ancestors evolved to walk with purpose, and the main purpose was foraging, ambling along looking for objects to eat, wear, use as tools, or make living space more comfortable. Sound familiar? Nowadays we call this "shopping." I believe it's a biological imperative.

In my work with overweight clients, I've found shopping to be far and away the most powerful walk motivator. With malls virtually everywhere, you can walk miles while window-shopping even in the dead of a Midwest winter or a desert summer. So if you love to shop, you're holding an exercise ace. An ideal C-level workout for you would be meandering through a mall or home-improvement center, looking at handbags or power tools or whatever else floats your boat. On each workout walk, you can purchase a 4-day win reward—a pen if you don't have much money, a Mercedes if you do. But the ambling itself is the real point.

If you don't like to window-shop, spend the next days observing the activities that keep you on your feet at home or work. If you're a Martha Stewart type who enjoys organizing objects, weeding the garden, or harvesting apples, go for it—and remember, a heavy ankle bracelet on each leg makes for an even better workout! (No offense, Ms. Stewart. I think that whole prison thing was an outrage.) Whatever your preferred walking activity, buy a pedometer (they cost between $5 and $30) and for 4 days, record your number of daily steps. Then take 100 more steps a day for days, another 100 for the next days, and so on.

MY FAVORITE WALKING WAYS

Please write down three or more activities you enjoy that require walking.

_____

_____

_____

_____

WORKOUT B: SLOW BURN

"Slow burn" is my term for a workout that stirs your blood and burns calories but doesn't break down a lot of muscle tissue (which intense exercise is meant to do so that the muscle will grow back stronger). Workout B requires that you do something active enough to make you breathe a bit harder and sweat more than you do while puttering around the house or mall. Choose a sport or fitness activity you like, then use any resource, from a paid coach or trainer to an exercise class to a book or magazine, to pinpoint a workout that appeals to you.

Your B-level workout should push you to about 50 percent of your maximum athletic capacity for 30 minutes to an hour. That means that you never quite become too breathless to talk while exercising (except during brief periods, when you're running the bases or doing your 20th pushup) and that you quit well before any of your muscles get to the point of fatigue failure. You should finish the exercise session feeling peppier and more fired up than when you started.

This is the time to start doing activities you've always wanted to try. I've seen overweight clients who've never been active start with D workouts, progress to C workouts, then suddenly realize they can do B-level workouts they thought they'd never experience: salsa dancing, kayaking, waterskiing, martial arts, rock climbing, hiding in trees from the police.

MY FAVORITE SLOW-BURN ACTIVITIES

Write down three or more types of physical exercise you've enjoyed in your life or an activity you haven't tried that looks like it might be fun.

_____

_____

_____

_____

WORKOUT A: ALL-OUT EFFORT

If you already exercise, all-out effort means the workout you think you should do every day but usually don't. There's a term to describe people who go all out all the time. That term is "injured." When I'm healthy, relaxed, not traveling, and getting plenty of sleep, I can handle an all-out workout every 3 days. Beyond that, I see signs of overtraining: waking up tired, having an elevated resting pulse rate, losing enthusiasm for exercise, feeling achy all over, and wanting to smack people. If you start noticing these symptoms, you need to take some minimum days or at the very least dial down a notch to a B-, C-, or D-level workout.

That said, jump in and identify ways you love going all out. Many of my clients like dancing, power yoga, cycling (outside or in a spin class), and hiking, as well as gym-based training. Load-bearing exercise, where your body has to carry its own weight or some other heavy item such as a backpack or your spouse, has lots of benefits. Among other things, it creates more muscle, which raises your metabolism, and helps prevent osteoporosis. So even if your favorite sport is swimming, throw in some weight-bearing exercise every few workouts.

Remember, *you never have to go all out to be physically fit and naturally thin.* Once you've worked your way through D-, C-, and B-level workouts, going all out occasionally is a blast. It will fill your brain and body with endorphins and other endogenous opioids—you'll get the famous "runner's high," which is literally like a big dose of free, legal morphine. But all-out effort is the icing; the cake is everyday trudging around. If you train like Adam rather than Caroline, you'll get high a lot.

MY FAVORITE ALL-OUT EFFORTS

Write down three or more ways you might enjoy an all-out exercise session.

_____

_____

_____

_____

If you're already on an exercise program that you enjoy, fine, continue it. But for the next 4 days, gather data about your own physical-action preferences from the small and inconspicuous to the large and dramatic. When you get to action, you'll be working out for a minimum of 15 minutes on every day that is not a minimum day. That may mean simply standing up and shifting your weight from foot to foot while you're on the phone with your mom, or it may mean cycling the Tour de France. By creating different options and always staying in a zone that's both innately enjoyable and geared to match your energy on any given day, you'll become one of those people who stays perpetually active without burning out. You may end up in a thousand-dollar gym outfit, but even if you're just shadow dancing in your bedroom, you'll have all the right moves.

"Choose New Moves"
4-Day Win

Ridiculously Easy Daily Goal: *Each day for the next 4 days, I'll observe and*

record my favorite ways to fidget, stroll about, do mild formal exercise, and go

physically all out. _____

Small Daily Reward: _____

_____

Slightly Larger 4-Day Reward: _____

_____

	Dates of My Current 4-Day Win	Check Off Completed Days Here
Day 1:	____ / ____ / ____	_____
Day 2:	____ / ____ / ____	_____
Day 3:	____ / ____ / ____	_____
Day 4:	____ / ____ / ____	_____

If you're already on a weight-loss regimen, remember that the 4-day win will enhance it, not conflict with it. If you know what to do, this program will help you do what you know. Feel free to stay on any weight-loss program while you learn 4-day win skills!

CHAPTER 28

PACKING YOUR PARACHUTE

PREPARATION CHECKLIST

Congratulations! After only a couple of hundred pages, you've reached the point where most diet books begin!

We've dwelt so heavily on the first three stages in the transtheoretical model of change because, although they're necessary to create lasting transformation, virtually no weight-loss books, magazines, or diet experts address them. Instead, all these authorities focus exclusively on the action phase. It's as though we have huge numbers of books on how to skydive that consider only the skill of actually leaping from the plane without even considering how to pack, position, or use a parachute.

Each time you've gone into weight-loss action without putting time and focus into pre-contemplation, contemplation, and preparation, your brain has become more deeply imprinted with famine reactions. Your body has been regeared to gain even more fat than you had before you started dieting. If you've done the 4-day wins that apply to your situation, on the other hand, you've prepared yourself for real change. You've set up not just one more diet but a new life, the life of a naturally thin person. In your past few 4-day wins, you've been assembling the information, equipment, and support people that will allow you to make this change. Now there's just one more exercise to do before this final prep-check.

EXPLANATION: PACKING YOUR PARACHUTE

There's one very important category of information you need to have right at your fingertips: a resource list of nonfood nurturing items. You can make this list by identifying things that correspond with lean living on your fatness lifeline and with things that make you feel those Rat-Park sensations of being happily ensconced in a benevolent environment. These things are nourishing to your spirit. Identify as many of them as possible; they're your key to stopping emotional or comfort eating.

IDENTIFYING YOUR NONFOOD NURTURERS

Go back to Chapters 14 and 15. Note any activities or items that correlate with positive feelings and skinny habits. List 10 of these below:

1. _____   6. _____

2. _____   7. _____

3. _____   8. _____

4. _____   9. _____

5. _____   10. _____

Now supplement the list above by thinking of at least five items that fit in the following categories for you:

- *Enjoyable tactile experiences.* Sex ranks high on most people's list of favorite tactile experiences, but all forms of comfortable touch are powerfully nourishing to the human body and soul. Being touched or even petting the cat triggers the same endogenous opioids that you produce when you eat buttery, sugary, or savory things. If you do any comfort eating, replacing it with tactile pleasure is a superb idea. Massages, spa treatments, manicures, even getting a haircut can be wonderfully nourishing. If there are no other warm-blooded beings available for pawing, try another sensory experience like a hot bath or shower, silk or flannel sheets, fuzzy socks . . . you get the idea.

11. _____

12. _____

13. _____

14. _____

15. _____

- *Info-fun.* Learning things about topics that interest you is another way to nourish yourself. This is not value-added learning, like memorizing tax forms or studying something you should know. I like learning about brain function and behavioral biology, which is why I'm writing this book. But learning about a celebrity's latest divorce is every bit as valid a nonfood nurturer if it's really absorbing for you. What do you love to learn?

16. _____

17. _____

18. _____

19. _____

20. _____

- *Being with beings.* There are certain people who drain your energy and others who feed it—without food. Make a list of the people who fill your soul. Pets count, too. Some of my favorite people are authors I've never met: They nurture me through their books. I have other friends who never existed except as fictional characters in movies. Certain TV personalities feel like personal friends. Spending time with any of these folks, through any form of communication, nourishes.

21. _____

22. _____

23. _____

24. _____

25. _____

These and any other nonfood nurturers you enjoy will be a crucial part of the parachute you'll need as you leap from the airplane of your old life into the wide-open spaces of your new one, dealing with the stiff wind of old habits as you watch the hard cold ground of rebound weight gain rushing ever nearer—until you pull the ripcord of 4-day win skills you've been learning and practicing while reading this book so that you float happily through the sunny skies of weight loss, attempting not to land in the Doberman Attack Dog Farm of people who will want to have carnal relations with you as your body gets ever nearer to perfection.

Now, go through the following checklist. Cross off any items you won't be needing (some people need exercise equipment or special food, others don't). Then, over the next 4 days, make sure you have every object, piece of information, or arrangement for logistical support that you need to start your new life.

EXERCISE: LIFE LAUNCH PREPARATION CHECKLIST

Cross out anything you won't need, then check off each item as you compile it. In addition to the items you've listed in the blanks above, you may need . . .

_____ Books, magazines, or other literature specifying your favorite healthy-eating diet

_____ Membership in Jenny Craig, Weight Watchers, or other weight-loss program

_____ Information on diet classes, Overeaters Anonymous meetings, or other instructional program

_____ Established relationship with coach, trainer, diet buddy, or other support people

_____ Righteous food (whatever your diet requires) in appropriate quantities

_____ Wicked food in profuse abundance (may be kept by a friend if necessary)

_____ Books, articles, and Web site information describing your chosen exercise program

_____ Exercise equipment

_____ Workout clothing (get good shoes!)

_____ Workout log (so you can fill out your 4-day wins)

_____ Relationship with exercise buddy (appointments for exercise set up)

_____ List of knowledgeable helpers you can turn to for fitness advice (doctors, trainers, dietitians, coaches, etc.)

_____ Membership at a gym, dance studio, yoga center, or other exercise location

READY, SET . . .

If you have everything you need to support the new you—a slender, healthy, vibrant, energetic person with more admirers than the Eiffel Tower—it's finally time to move into action. Long before you cracked this book, you had the necessry facts and comprehension to lose weight.

All along, you've known what to do. Now it's time to do what you know.

"Life Launch Prep Check"
4-Day Win

Ridiculously Easy Daily Goal: _Within the next 4 days, I'll compile all the_

information, objects, and appointments necessary to start my new lifestyle, one in

which I'll eat less, move more, and be so fit and healthy all will envy me to the

limits of the galaxy. _____

Small Daily Reward: _____

_____

Slightly Larger 4-Day Reward: _____

_____

	Dates of My Current 4-Day Win	**Check Off Completed Days Here**
Day 1:	___ / ___ / ___	_____
Day 2:	___ / ___ / ___	_____
Day 3:	___ / ___ / ___	_____
Day 4:	___ / ___ / ___	_____

If you're already on a weight-loss regimen, remember that the 4-day win will enhance it, not conflict with it. If you know what to do, this program will help you do what you know. Feel free to stay on any weight-loss program while you learn 4-day win skills!

STAGE
4

ACTION

CHAPTER 29

CREATING YOUR DAYMAP

THE SECOND MOST IMPORTANT WEIGHT-LOSS SKILL IN THE HISTORY OF THE UNIVERSE

When my son was 2 weeks old, I attended a seminar for parents of children with disabilities. That's when I realized that compared to many things that can go wrong with a newborn, Adam's Down syndrome was a veritable walk in the park. There were about 20 other adults at the seminar, many with infants in their arms, all with shell-shocked expressions on their faces. A lot of the babies had unusual accessories: stomach-access feeding tubes, oxygen masks, bandages. I've seen jollier crowds at race riots.

The seminar teacher began by telling us all that the reason we felt so rotten wasn't because of our babies, but because life had confronted us with an unexpected set of changes—big ones.

"People resist changing habitual patterns," he explained.

Then he asked us to guess what single action was statistically likely to add the most years to our lifespan. The answer? Not giving up sugar, fat, cigarettes, or booze; not meditating or doing yoga; not exercising. The answer is boringly simple: fastening your seatbelt. After revealing this, the teacher asked how many of the participants had fastened their seatbelts that very morning. I was surprised when only five people raised their hands (I was lucky; I had a car with passive restraints, so I got credit for wearing my belt).

"Okay," said the teacher. "Now you know that this one behavior, which takes about 3 seconds when you get into a car, is more likely to lengthen your life than any other single behavior. Tomorrow, on your way here, fasten your seatbelts."

The next day, when all of us had re-congregated, the teacher asked for another show of hands. Who had remembered to fasten their seatbelts? Out of the 15 people who hadn't worn their belts the day before, only one had remembered to add this small action to her daily routine.

"How much motivation do we need," said the teacher, "to make one tiny, simple change? Apparently, more than longer lives. *People resist changing habitual patterns.*"

For those of us who wish to avoid becoming statistics in stories about the Obesity Crisis, this is one of those bad-news, good-news things. It means that making significant changes in our eating and/or exercise patterns is not nearly as easy as most fitness books imply. But it also means that if we *can* make changes, and sustain them long enough to make them "habitual patterns," we'll keep doing them come hell or high water, just because we're used to them.

This is where 4-day wins really prove their mettle. Though it takes five linked wins (a total of 20 days) to make something truly habitual, an action will stop feeling different and strange if we can hang in there and repeat it, preferably at the same time of day, for 4 days. This is the transformative power of circadian rhythm, which is the basic reason 4-day wins work.

EXPLANATION: CIRCADIAN RHYTHM

"Circadian" literally means "around the day." Our bodies are designed to repeat certain functions at approximately 24-hour intervals. Now that we've reached the "action" stage of your weight-loss process, we're going to use this phenomenon to make healthy living habitual for you. This, according to my highly scientific ranking method of reflecting upon the experience of my clients and my ownself, is the Second Most Important Weight-Loss Skill in the History of the Universe.

Some circadian rhythms, such as sleep patterns, are quite resistant to change. For example, some of us are natural night owls. We feel most zippy as evening comes on, work well in the dark, and fall asleep between midnight and 3 a.m. Others are "morning people," who head for dreamland by

9 p.m. and are rarin' to get-up-and-go by 5 in the morning. I think I speak for all us night owls when I say to morning people: We are so impressed by all the things you do before sunrise, and if you don't stop that cheery whistling, we will drag ourselves out of bed one morning just long enough to beat you with a frying pan. I have tried my whole life to become a morning person, and so have all my biological relatives, and as God is our witness, it can't be done without chemical assistance.

Eating also follows circadian patterns. Say you're used to picking up a Bacon 'n' Butter Biscuit from your favorite truck stop every morning at 8. One night you go to a village feast and consume way too much mead and wild boar. Because your body's metabolism becomes more efficient at night—even if you stay awake—a lot of those mead-and-boar calories, which would be burned off if you ate them during the day, are stored as fat. Nevertheless, the next morning at about 8, you'll find yourself headed for the truck stop, tummy rumbling for your Bacon 'n' Butter Biscuit. Your body expects its daily treat at the usual time, even though it doesn't need calories as much as it does on a typical morning. This is one way misuse of circadian rhythm can make you fat, and a lot of us do it all the time.

The good news is that it's much easier to manipulate food-related circadian rhythms than sleep cycles. In fact, they can be one of your most powerful allies in taking off weight and staying lean. It takes 4 days of consistent practice to establish a circadian eating pattern. However, remember that people resist even tiny, highly motivated change, like seatbelt-fastening. Eating less and moving more are big changes that affect us at the most primal level. Establishing an effective circadian change—one that won't result in white-knuckling and backlash bingeing—must happen gradually. In fact, you're more likely to lose weight if you establish your ideal circadian rhythm before beginning to eat less and move more.

This means that your first action step, before starting either a new diet or exercise program, should be to establish daily activity patterns that support your new healthy lifestyle. Whatever your choice of programs, the most important determinant of whether you can stay on them is where you are physically located at a given time on a typical day. In other words, you will lose or gain weight, get more or less fit, depending on your daily habitual schedule. I call this your "daymap." Observing your daymap, then changing it 4 days at a time, is the key action that will transform your body forever.

EXERCISE: MAKING A DAYMAP

A daymap is a way of charting your physical location and activities during a 24-hour period. In this exercise, you'll learn to make one. You're simply going to draw a circle with points around it, like numbers on a clock, that show where you were, what you were doing there, and how long you stayed in that place, doing that thing.

You start making a daymap by writing down the place and time period you spent sleeping last night. At the top of a page (generally the 12 o'clock position on the "clock face" of your circle) write something like "11 p.m. to 7 a.m. In bed, asleep." Then write your next location and activity, along with the duration of the activity, at about the 1 o'clock position on the clock face. Continue noting your location, activities, and their duration clockwise

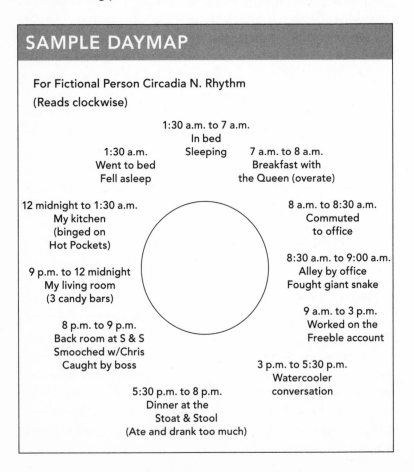

SAMPLE DAYMAP

For Fictional Person Circadia N. Rhythm
(Reads clockwise)

1:30 a.m. to 7 a.m.
In bed
Sleeping

1:30 a.m.
Went to bed
Fell asleep

7 a.m. to 8 a.m.
Breakfast with
the Queen (overate)

12 midnight to 1:30 a.m.
My kitchen
(binged on
Hot Pockets)

8 a.m. to 8:30 a.m.
Commuted
to office

9 p.m. to 12 midnight
My living room
(3 candy bars)

8:30 a.m. to 9:00 a.m.
Alley by office
Fought giant snake

8 p.m. to 9 p.m.
Back room at S & S
Smooched w/Chris
Caught by boss

9 a.m. to 3 p.m.
Worked on the
Freeble account

5:30 p.m. to 8 p.m.
Dinner at the
Stoat & Stool
(Ate and drank too much)

3 p.m. to 5:30 p.m.
Watercooler
conversation

around the circle until you've accounted for your 24-hour day. It's especially important to note times you ate, and whether that eating was healthy or excessive. Also note times you exercised, formally or informally. Your complete daymap might look something like this:

As you can see, during this 24-hour period, daymap-maker Circadia N. Rhythm overate at breakfast, snacked on candy when stressed, and binged at night. The only thing during her day that could count as exercise is fighting the giant snake, which is obviously not an everyday occurrence (usually, she fights a giant spider). Circadia sleeps only 5½ hours at night, which isn't enough for most people. If she wants to become healthier and lose weight, she'll have to subtract some unhealthy food, reduce stress, and add exercise and sleep to her daily activity mix. To change her unhealthy patterns, Circadia first has to notice them, seeing them from her Watcher identity, which is why daymaps are so helpful.

LOOKING FOR CIRCADIAN PATTERNS

Obviously, every day is different for each of us. It's very rare for me to have two similar days in a row; I'm constantly traveling, meeting new people, and doing odd things. Even so, there are circadian patterns that show up in my daymaps—things I do consistently at more or less the same time, almost every day. These *circadian patterns are the access points for changing your lifestyle in ways that will make you a thin person.* These are the times and places to implement your preferred ways of eating less and moving more.

To begin seeing circadian patterns, you have to make multiple daymaps—and I'll give you one guess how many days I want you to map out for starters. That's right: four. Let's say Circadia makes four consecutive daymaps, and discovers that she overeats at breakfast every day, and binges at night three times. One other consistent pattern is that she spends the afternoon chatting by the watercooler with her friends at work. Circadia could choose any of these patterns as access points for changing her life (you'll find detailed instructions for doing this in the next two chapters). For example, she could eat a sensible breakfast, then follow up with 10 minutes of quiet meditation, going to her inner Watcher, observing her emotions, questioning her own anxiety-producing thoughts. Instead of just standing by the watercooler all afternoon, she could shift from foot to foot, or even pace, and burn off hundreds more calories.

GETTING THE 4-DAY FACTS

By tracking your daymap for 4 consecutive days, without changing anything, you'll begin to get a feel for the circadian patterns in your own eating
and exercise routine—not the routine you *should* have, not the one you *mean
to* have, not necessarily the one you *think* you have, but the one you actually
do have. Studies show that we remember things we *want* to remember, and
fuzz details we don't like. That's why so many weekend warriors see themselves as "daily" exercisers. It's why one woman told me with a completely
straight face, "I stick to my eating program absolutely, except for a few cookies at work, but those shouldn't count" (she was getting about 1,000 calories
a day in cookies alone).

For your next 4-day win, I'd like you to make daymaps that track your
location, activity, and eating/drinking as they actually occur. Please don't
judge yourself or fudge on the facts; we're not doing this to show how bad
you are, or to take away your daily pleasures and turn your life into an iron
cage of value-added, zero-calorie rules. On the contrary, I want you to accept
and enjoy the circadian rhythms that *really, truly* make your life feel joyful
and abundant. Then we're going to tweak those rhythms, just a little, so that
your typical day includes the eating and activity patterns that will make you
feel and look awesome.

"Observing My Daymap"
4-Day Win

Ridiculously Easy Daily Goal: _Within the next 4 days, I'll track my daily_

activities on a "daymap," showing where I was at any given time of day, and

what I was doing there. I'll devote particular attention to times and places where

I ate and exercised, and how much sleep I got.

Small Daily Reward: _____

_____

Slightly Larger 4-Day Reward: _____

_____

	Dates of My Current 4-Day Win	**Check Off Completed Days Here**
Day 1:	____/____/____	_____
Day 2:	____/____/____	_____
Day 3:	____/____/____	_____
Day 4:	____/____/____	_____

If you're already on a weight-loss regimen, remember that the 4-day win will enhance it, not conflict with it. If you know what to do, this program will help you do what you know. Feel free to stay on any weight-loss program while you learn 4-day win skills!

CHAPTER 30

"MOVE MORE" DAYMAP ADJUSTMENT

EDGING INTO EXERCISE

One of my all-time favorite clients was a professional baseball player I'll call Dan, who was making the transition from athletics to civilian life. Dan was an impressive specimen in every way: smart, funny, energetic, and incredibly fit. At the time he consulted me, I was doing a lot of my usual traveling and public speaking. Between my erratic scheduling, sleep loss, lack of access to healthy food, and adrenal burnout, I'd gained several pounds and fallen off all the various wagons of healthy eating and exercise habits. I kept meaning to cut back on the flan and get back to regular exercise, but I never seemed to find the time or energy. Then one day, when we were talking about his baseball career, Dan tossed out an offhand comment that would change my muscle tone forever.

"Ninety percent of being in shape," he said, "is getting to the gym."

For me it was, as Oprah might say, a lightbulb moment. Right then and there, I decided that I would re-establish a pattern of going to the gym—not *doing* anything at the gym, just *getting* there. So the next day, I dropped off my kids at school and drove directly to the gym, where I parked my car, listened to a song on my favorite radio station, started the car again, and went home. The next day I did the same thing . . . and the next . . . and the next.

By the 4th day, my new daymap pattern came very easily—my brain and body *expected* to drive to the gym after taking the kids to school. Then I knew I could safely up the ante—*a little*. For the next 4 days, after arriving at the gym, I went in and pedaled a stationary bike for approximately 3 minutes, just long enough to listen to another favorite song on my MP3 player. My next 4-day win consisted of increasing my pedaling sessions to 7 minutes (two songs). When that felt habitual, I added one round of circuit training with light weight to my cycling routine (I bought a few new tunes from the Internet as a reward).

After the third 4-day win, something rather dramatic happened. I'd been increasing my workout by tiny increments, but suddenly, my body took over and decided it *loved* the gym. I no longer needed a reward for showing up and exercising; in fact, I felt edgy and disappointed if I didn't get a chance to lift weights (please remember, I'd previously chosen this form of exercise because I find it inherently enjoyable). Despite the chaos of my schedule, my sometimes-crippling autoimmune disease, and my utter athletic ineptitude, I'm now something of a gym rat.

Whatever your preferred exercise, you can increase your own activity to healthy levels by using a similar 4-day win strategy. As your very first action on your 4-day win exercise program, I'd like you to modify your daymap so that you show up in an appropriate place to exercise, at approximately the same time, for 4 consecutive days. *What exercise you choose to do is less important than your arrival at the designated location.*

EXPLANATION: DAILY PRACTICE

I've worked with several professional musicians, and they've all told me that if you want to play a musical instrument, you're better off practicing for 15 minutes every day (less than 2 hours a week) than practicing for 6 hours every Sunday. By the same token, studies show that people who write for a few minutes every day produce better prose than those who wait for the muse to strike, then churn out pages and pages (the writing is judged by people who don't know which writer used which method). I'm not methodical by nature, and I hate repetition. Yet, even I benefit enormously from establishing daily circadian patterns in certain areas. Exercise is definitely one of these areas. Now that you've reached the "Action" stage of your weight-loss lifestyle, you'll be exercising every day.

FINDING THE EXERTION SWEET SPOT

How does my policy of exercising each and every day fit with my general torpidness and lack of discipline? You'll understand how if you review the chapters in this book that discuss adrenal burnout and choosing "new moves." To keep exercising every day, you need to hit a "sweet spot" between exerting too little, and exerting too much. *Exercising either too little or too much will cause you to end up in lousy shape.* So, start by looking realistically at your 4-day collection of "daymaps." How much are you already exercising? Not on a good day, when the kids are healthy and your deadlines are far away and you've had plenty of rest, but on a *real* day, when none of these things are true.

There have been whole years in my life when a "Minimum Day" was all I could realistically manage. During my three pregnancies, for example, my body reacted as though the fetuses I carried were badly-transplanted organs, so I was not only plagued by autoimmune problems, but violently nauseated and bizarrely weak. It was during these long, helpless stretches of time (each pregnancy seemed to last roughly as long as the Pleistocene Era) I realized that we can improve our physical health without moving at all. How? You've been learning how through this entire book.

Every time you access your Watcher self, delve into your treasure-chest of positive memories, or become the compassionate Watcher of your own pain (try all three at once!) your body chemistry changes for the better. In his book *Love and Survival,* Dr. Dean Ornish of Harvard presents a vast amount of data showing that the capacity to love and be loved has profound effects on things like heart disease and longevity—often more than diet and exercise. He also mentions that when he lectures on this topic, doctors get up and walk out in disgust, violently upset that he isn't sticking to the "empirical" realities of diet and exercise, instead of all that ridiculously accurate and convincing evidence that our best workout is stilling our minds and expanding our souls.

If you want to go a step further than exercising your emotional "heart," there's scientific evidence that suggests simply visualizing exercises can make your muscles stronger. Researchers at the Cleveland Clinic Foundation had a group of subjects *imagine* exercising either their little fingers or their biceps for 15 minutes, 5 times a week. The biceps group increased strength in that muscle by 13.4 percent. The little-finger group improved strength by 53 percent. (I picture them on the streets, threateningly flexing their Pinkies of Doom, intimidating gangbangers.) All of this is just more evidence that the brain-body connection means thought, as well as effort, should be involved in your fitness program.

So, no matter where your body is located, *your 4-day win workouts require you to spend your exercise time in the place of Thinner Peace.* If you're sick or injured, "going" to this inner place once a day, increasing your ability to calm yourself, and feeling a relaxation response is your whole workout. You'll feel that this is the "sweet spot" of exertion for you—the place at the edge of too hard, but not over it. Too little challenge, and your brain won't produce the dopamine surge that makes working out addictive. Too much challenge, and your body won't be able to supply the serotonin hit that transfers excitement over to contentment.

Experiment to see what level of workout feels best to you—almost difficult, but ultimately very satisfying. If you're only capable of a D workout, such as pacing or fidgeting, just do it in a designated spot (my D workout used to consist of lying down on the family-room floor amidst my rug rats, and stretching for 15 minutes). If a C workout seems possible, go walking (in the mall, on the treadmill, through the neighbor's flowerbed—anything that makes you happy). A level B workout may involve showing up at the dance studio to meet with your class, or pushing yourself *a little* to go cross-country skiing. If you're a rabid exerciser who loves to go all-out, put on your cleats, helmet, body armor, and hip waders, and have a helicopter drop you into shark-infested water for a long-distance swim. Just make sure that every day, your daymap includes a "workout."

Here's how to know if your efforts to move more are too ambitious: they don't happen. You make all sorts of plans to start taking long power walks, or do hundreds of squat-thrusts in your basement, or bicycling to Lapland, but you never do them. The fix is always to reduce the intensity of your workouts. Back off a level, right down to meditation if that's all you can actually do. Sustain a lower-than-you-want level of exercise for 4 days. If you continue this, you'll soon experience . . .

TAKEOFF VELOCITY

Remember how I got to 10 minutes of cardio and a single circuit of light weights, then suddenly started working out much more intensely? I call this "takeoff velocity." It's actually a very common experience for the folks I've coached *who did their exercise 4-day wins according to instructions.* I believe it's because the "training effect" that makes our bodies stronger follows a geometric growth curve; very slow at first, slightly faster until you reach the phase called the "tipping point," and extremely rapid after that.

People who try too hard, too soon, or don't push themselves into the sweet spot on a regular schedule, never reach takeoff velocity. They're not willing to do the low-effort, slow-increase part of the process; but in trying to leap forward, they exhaust themselves quickly, having one negative exercise experience after another. By far the biggest problem I have with my clients is that they won't do *small* workouts. But as a creaky, battle-worn, athletically impaired, chronically ill, middle-aged woman who now has a blast doing a whole bunch of sports, I'm here to tell you that if you're willing to increase exercise slowly, starting with just going to a certain location and building very gradually from there, you'll come to enjoy living in your body more than you thought possible. Here are a couple of exercises to make this happen.

EXERCISES: WORKING IN WORKING OUT

Exercise 1: Reframing Your Workout as a Treat

The most common reason overweight people give for not exercising is that they don't have time. First of all, if you can't fit visualization or fidgeting into your schedule, you must be—no offense—deceased. Second, you may be blocking yourself from finding time because exercise has negative associations for you. I still descend into despondency and loathing any time I recall my 7th-grade physical education teacher. And that's not even mentioning the hideous trauma of changing clothes in a crowded locker room at a time in my life when I was so self-conscious about my chubby body that my ears frequently burst into flames.

Obviously, by choosing a variety of exercise options that you enjoy, and by connecting with people who motivate you, you create much more incentive to exercise than if you simply slog through a bunch of hated calisthenics. But there's a final barrier many people run into when it comes to altering their daymaps to include exercise. We put other people first—and second, and third, and fourth, and fifth—so that the time we might use window shopping or meditating or throwing the javelin gets devoured by service to others. "I should exercise," we think, but there's always something else we think we should do more. Write down all the reasons you should move more in the spaces below. Keep going until you run out of answers (use your own paper if necessary).

1. I should take time to exercise because _____

2. I should take time to exercise because _____

3. I should take time to exercise because _____

4. I should take time to exercise because _____

5. I should take time to exercise because _____

6. I should take time to exercise because _____

7. I should take time to exercise because _____

8. I should take time to exercise because _____

9. I should take time to exercise because _____

10. I should take time to exercise because _____

Read through all these statements and notice how you feel about exercise, and your whole life, as you hold them in your mind. Got it? Okay. Now, shake all that out of your head and finish the following sentence fragment, again, in as many different ways as you can.

1. I deserve time to exercise because _____

2. I deserve time to exercise because _____

3. I deserve time to exercise because _____

4. I deserve time to exercise because _____

5. I deserve time to exercise because _____

6. I deserve time to exercise because _____

256

7. I deserve time to exercise because _____

8. I deserve time to exercise because _____

9. I deserve time to exercise because _____

10. I deserve time to exercise because _____

Read over this list, and you'll probably get a much more accurate image of your life's realities. Exercise that's chosen to match your tastes, motivated by people you enjoy, and tailor-made for your current level of fitness, *is way more fun than just sitting still.*

Exercise 2: Commiting to Your First "Move More" 4-Day Win

Now that you've done all the preparation, chosen an activity that you'll enjoy without getting exhausted, and set up circumstances that motivate you, it's time to make moving more part of your circadian pattern. Find a place on your existing daymap where you might work in 15 minutes of exercise. Remember, this could be 15 minutes of visualizing, fidgeting, walking, or hanging out with a personal trainer. Shoot for the level of workout one notch *lower* than what seems reasonable. Then, stay in the place where you'll be exercising, *without increasing your physical exercise at all,* for 4 days.

On your second "move more" 4-day win, add 5 minutes of exercise. Do not exceed this limit for 4 days. Then up the amount of exercise again, by 5–10 minutes. If you ever feel achy, insomniacal, exhausted after exercising, or just generally drained, move your workout level down a notch—*but keep your appointment with your body, even if this only means creating a relaxation response for 15 minutes.* After a few linked 4-day wins, you'll probably notice an abrupt increase in your enjoyment and enthusiasm for exercising. Once you have five linked 4-day wins (if you've stayed well within your physical tolerance), you'll have a brand new habit—and remember, people hate breaking habitual patterns. You won't be an out-of-shape person who's trying to act like an athlete. You'll be an athlete who vaguely remembers a bygone time when exercise wasn't fun. Stay alert to your own physical cues and sensations, and this is the person you'll be for the rest of your (considerably lengthened) life.

"Edging Into Exercise" 4-Day Win

Ridiculously Easy Daily Goal: *For the next 4 days, I'll go to a place where*

I plan to exercise at approximately the same time every day. If I am excited about

exercising, I'll do it. But I'll still get my 4-day reward for just showing up, or for

a D-level workout like fidgeting, if I'm not frisky enough to do a lot of exercise.

Small Daily Reward: _____

_____

Slightly Larger 4-Day Reward: _____

_____

	Dates of My Current 4-Day Win	**Check Off Completed Days Here**
Day 1:	___ / ___ / ___	_____
Day 2:	___ / ___ / ___	_____
Day 3:	___ / ___ / ___	_____
Day 4:	___ / ___ / ___	_____

If you're already on a weight-loss regimen, remember that the 4-day win will enhance it, not conflict with it. If you know what to do, this program will help you do what you know. Feel free to stay on any weight-loss program while you learn 4-day win skills!

CHAPTER 31

EATING DAYMAP ADJUSTMENT

FEEDING YOUR SOUL

Of all the many surprises my body has sprung on me, one of the weirdest has got to be lactation. My first child was born between my undergraduate and graduate programs at Harvard, when I saw myself basically as a computer with cellulite. And then, the day after delivering a baby, my body began delivering . . . milk! My mind had been in a state of denial about the fact that I was a mammal; now my chest rivaled the state of Wisconsin in exporting dairy products. I was (and please know I'm being forced to write this by the Citizens for the Merciless Use of Stupid Puns) udderly amazed.

Lactation also showed me how tightly our bodies replicate circadian patterns that control eating and appetite. If a nursing baby gets extra hungry at, say, noon on Thursday, the mother's body has trouble keeping up with demand, and the baby has to suckle more vigorously. In response, mom's mammary glands will increase production of milk by exactly the right amount at just about noon on Friday. If the baby wants less milk for dinner, the mother's body diminishes the supply in about 24 hours. Since we lactators need food to produce milk, during my nursing days I could feel my own appetite rise or fall in precise amounts, depending on how much nutrition my babies needed at a given time of day.

After all my little ones were weaned, I found I could still feel and use circadian patterns to influence what, when, and how much my body wanted to eat. In the last chapter, I advised you to use your body's circadian rhythm to develop habitual patterns of moving more. This skill is even more crucial when it comes to the most important element of any weight-loss strategy:

eating less. There are two strategies that will help you stick to whatever healthy-eating program you've chosen: daymap adjustment, and a process I call "SIN," short for "Substituting Inedible Nourishment." Here's how they're going to work for you.

EXPLANATION: YOUR APPETITE'S CIRCADIAN RHYTHM

Unlike sleep patterns, appetite patterns are easy to manipulate. If you eat 500 calories at noon today, your body will urge you—mildly at first—to eat 500 calories the following day, right around noon. Repeat the pattern for 4 days, and on the fifth day your body will assert it very clearly: "I want 500 calories, and I want it at noon, dammit!" At that point you can make another change—go ahead and eat at noon, but only have 400 calories. Your body will feel a little hungry and unfulfilled that first day, but the next day, if you eat 400 calories at noon, you'll feel a bit less hungry and disappointed. Persist for 2 more days, and your appetite will have learned to tell you, "I want 400 calories at noon!"

Please notice that we're talking about actual physical appetite—body reactions, not mind reactions. But as we've seen, much of our eating (if we're overweight, *most* of our eating) is driven by mental and emotional hunger, not gut hunger. This is where SIN comes in. "Substituting Inedible Nourishment" means giving yourself something to feed mind- or heart-hunger every time you reduce the amount of food you're tucking into your tummy. I've said this before, and I'll say it again, because so many of my clients ignore it—to their regret. *You have to increase some form of nourishment that isn't food, at the time you're used to eating, to successfully reduce the amount of food you eat.*

BALANCING YOUR NOURISHMENT EQUATION

When my overweight clients go on diets, they always pledge to live as righteous Puritans. Instead of eating that extra bagel at 3 p.m., they're going to do 100 situps or walk a mile in the snow. In other words, they try to substitute hardship for pleasure and comfort. *This doesn't work.* To lose weight, you'll be reducing the amount of comfort you get from food. *If you want this to be a gentle, permanent process rather than a violent and temporary one, you must provide yourself with enough non-edible nourishment to balance the pleasure and contentment you'll no longer be getting from stuffing your face.*

For example, a few weeks ago I noticed that I was eating breakfast for a long, long time. I'd finish a reasonable meal, then start rooting around for other things to eat. I'd continue munching until I was uncomfortably full, but even so, it was hard to stop. When I realized this, I went into my Watcher mind and mentally replayed a breakfast binge, just as I've advised you to do when you can't stop eating (see Chapter 10).

From my Watcher perspective, I could see the problem. My daymap pattern was to get up, eat breakfast, and then go to work writing stuff and checking e-mail. Now, writing can be enjoyable for me if I get into a certain zone, but most of the time, I experience it as a grinding task. However, I vastly prefer it to checking e-mail, which is about as much fun for me as being pecked to death by ducks (I get hundreds a day, most unsolicited). So each morning I was waking up to a pleasant experience (breakfast!) then trying to stop the fun and plunge directly into aversive tasks. In other words, when breakfast ended, life got very difficult. So my Wild Child self was making sure breakfast never ended.

The fix for this was very simple, once I'd recognized the problem. I had to SIN (Substitute Inedible Nourishment) at the point in my daymap where I was overeating. Fortunately, I have a long list of non-food nourishers (just like the ones I made you list in Chapter 26 as part of "packing your parachute"). I changed my daymap by throwing in a little SIN right after breakfast. Now, my pattern is to eat a nutritious breakfast, go directly to a spot on my comfiest couch where I have a view of my favorite wind sculpture, and spend 15 minutes looking through one of my gazillion how-to books on art. Drawing and painting are two of my most compelling SINs, so this truly feeds my heart and soul. As soon as I implemented this SIN, the compulsion to overeat at breakfast disappeared. But I know that if I stop SINning, I'll overeat again.

THE BEST DIET DRUGS EVER—FREE!

Substituting Inedible Nourishment is especially vital because it keeps your brain from going into a famine reaction. Suppose you eat your yummy Jenny Craig lunch, then find yourself feeling a little hungry and a lot sad about the fact that you're not supposed to eat again for a couple of hours. At this point, if you force yourself to run a mile, your body will assume there's some sort of food shortage, along with hungry predators, in your immediate neighborhood. You'll start pumping out the adrenaline, cortisol, and glucocorticoids that are triggered by a hunger and fear, and your brain will become even more likely to crave huge portions of cheesecake.

On the other hand, if you follow up your Jenny Craig meal by spending 15 minutes cuddled up in an easy chair, petting your cat, and vividly recalling moments when you've felt pure love, you'll activate the parts of your brain that register rest, gentle touch, appreciation, and gratitude. Instead of stress hormones, you'll produce more oxytocin (the hormone that rules lactation, incidentally) and endogenous opioids. It's like a dose of free, legal, healthy morphine. This teaches your brain to relax the pressure to eat, and let go of stored fat instead of adding more. It improves your immune function, your cardiovascular health, your mood, and your trust in the goodness of the universe. SIN is the opposite of sinful, but it feels wickedly good.

EXERCISE: CHANGING YOUR EATING DAYMAP

Before you start changing your eating patterns, make sure that you assemble the information and supplies you wrote down in your "preparation checklist" from Chapter 26, plus your daymaps. Make sure you've listed lots of non-food nurturing items and activities in your mind or (preferably) in a notebook. Review the 4-day win skills you've learned throughout this book, especially those involved in "Contemplation." Then it's time to start changing your body's expectations about how much it will eat, and when.

STEP ONE: BEGIN CHANGING YOUR EATING DAYMAP BY SETTING A "CALORIE CURFEW"

Just as I advised you to begin go to your place of exercise at a certain time each day, I'd like you to *change your eating schedule before deliberately trying to reduce your calorie intake*. You'll start by creating a "curfew" on eating or drinking anything but water, which you can have all day, any day.

Even for night owls like me, or folks who work graveyard shifts and sleep all day, human metabolic circadian rhythms "turn down" the burning of calories at night. You'll be able to lose more weight more quickly if you eat when your metabolism is high (during the day) than if you eat when it's turned down (during the night).

It's essential to move back your curfew gradually. For example, if you're used to having a bedtime snack of cranberry crumpets at 11 p.m., right before going to bed, suddenly imposing a 7 p.m. curfew would be too drastic for you—it might trigger a famine reaction, get you into a pattern of binge-ing, and end up putting on fat, which would be a massive bummer for some-one with a massive bum. Push back curfew just half an hour, eating your crumpets at 10:30, for 4 days. Please note: I'm not telling you you can't have the crumpets, I'm just asking you to eat them a bit earlier.

STEP TWO: PUT A LITTLE SIN WHERE YOUR EVENING SNACK HAS BEEN

The first time you move back your eating curfew to 10:30, your body will get a little anxious. At 11, it might start telling you it wants more crumpets, because 11 is when it's used to getting them. So indulge in a little SIN. Read a good book, watch something fun on TV, page through a fashion magazine and plan the outfit you're going to buy for yourself as a 4-day win reward.

For women, anything touch-based, from a hot bath to hot sex, is an excellent SIN, since touch kick-starts those lovely endogenous opioids. By comparison, men are less attuned to touch, and much more attuned to visual stimuli. They also produce testosterone to balance their oxytocin, and tes-tosterone fuels erotic responses. So if you're a guy, sex is a particularly effec-tive substitute for a midnight snack, especially if you leave the lights on.

STEP THREE: KEEP MOVING BACK YOUR CURFEW UNTIL IT'S AT LEAST 3 HOURS EARLIER THAN BEDTIME

Generally, it's a good idea to stop eating after 7 or 8 p.m., depending on how late you stay up. Move back your latest meal of the day, half an hour at a time, until you no longer get hungry for 3 hours before bedtime.

PREPARING FOR THE BIG KAHUNA: EATING LESS, FOREVER

When you read the words "eating less, forever," do you feel any negative emotions? Does the phrase make you sad, angry, hopeless, or fearful? Does it make you want to binge? If so, watch your feelings and thoughts as the compassionate observer, and assure both sides of yourself—the Wild Child and the Dictator—that life is about to become richer, more abundant, more nourishing, and more fulfilling, not less.

Everything you've learned from this book is going to help you do one thing evolution never expected you'd have to do: sit peacefully in an environment overflowing with addictive, fattening food, and eat precisely the right types and amounts of food to be optimally healthy. You were born with this skill. As a tiny baby, you knew exactly how much milk to drink at each meal, and you stopped eating when you were satisfied. Nature, and perhaps your mother's newly multitasking breasts, knew exactly how to feed you. Your appetite and food supply balanced perfectly, without conscious effort, steely willpower, intellectual knowledge, diet books, or an aggressively helpful personal trainer in Spandex shorts.

It's time to go back to that.

"Food Curfew" 4-Day Win

Ridiculously Easy Daily Goal: *For the next 4 days, I'll set a curfew on food consumption—in other words, I won't eat after (your time goes here). I'll substitute inedible nourishers to replace the comfort I once got from eating at that time.*

Small Daily Reward: _____

_____

Slightly Larger 4-Day Reward: _____

_____

	Dates of My Current 4-Day Win	Check Off Completed Days Here
Day 1:	____ / ____ / ____	_____
Day 2:	____ / ____ / ____	_____
Day 3:	____ / ____ / ____	_____
Day 4:	____ / ____ / ____	_____

If you're already on a weight-loss regimen, remember that the 4-day win will enhance it, not conflict with it. If you know what to do, this program will help you do what you know. Feel free to stay on any weight-loss program while you learn 4-day win skills!

CHAPTER 32

I WILL FIGHT NO MORE (AND EAT A BIT LESS) FOREVER

ACTUALLY LOSING WEIGHT

If you're a Jump-Start plan reader, you've seen this chapter already
Give it a gander and see how much more easily you can modify
your eating now that you've learned more Thinner Peace strategies.
Go, go, go!

The Pima Indians of Gila Valley, close to my own Arizona home, have a hell of a time losing weight. Of course, this wasn't true for most of the 2,000 years the Pima inhabited Gila Valley. As desert farmers, they ate native plants like squash and beans, and low-fat meat from rabbits and birds. They also underwent many periods of famine, and so (according to some researchers) the Pima experienced a lot of selective pressure that favored a so-called "thrifty gene" (the human leptin receptor gene is a prime suspect). This gene helped their bodies store fat very quickly in times of plenty, so as to live through times of want.

Then, in the 1920s, the natural water supply flowing through the Gila Valley was diverted for use by farmers who were not of Pima origin (three guesses which racial group these interlopers represented). To keep the Pima from starving in their now-permanently drought-stricken homeland, the

U.S. government began giving the tribe food, such as lard, cheese, and white flour. The results were disastrous. Today, at least half of the adults in the Gila Valley Pima community are obese, and 80 percent of those people have Type II diabetes.

Dr. Eric Ravussin has been studying the Pima since 1984. At one point, he trekked to a remote part of the Sierra Madre mountains in Mexico to visit a group of Pima who have the same genetic profile as the Arizona group, but live and eat in more traditional ways. The Mexican Pima studied by Dr. Ravussin weren't overweight, and only three had diabetes. His conclusion? "[I]f the Pima Indians of Arizona could return to some of their traditions, including a high degree of physical activity and a diet with less fat and more starch, we might be able to reduce the rate, and surely the severity, of unhealthy weight in most of the population,"

In other words, even if your genetic deck is stacked against you, it's still very possible to be lean and healthy if you (here it comes) eat less, move more. Surprise, surprise.

EXPLANATION: THE BOTTOM LINE FOR KEEPING YOUR BOTTOM IN LINE

I mention the Pima because their experience points out that people really do have distinctly, even dramatically different hereditary tendencies when it comes to getting fat. There are about 340 genes involved in determining your weight, and only identical siblings share exactly the same genetic profile, including its specific tendencies to be chubbier or leaner. Even if you don't have Pima ancestry, there are probably lots of people in the world who really can eat more than you do, while exercising less, and still be skinny.

This is not fair.

It is absolutely not fair. It is terribly, hideously, inexcusably unfair. It is so unfair that the government, the pope, the army, and God omnipotent really should do something to change it . . . which is probably what a bunch of people who starved to death in the Middle Ages thought about your ancestors being able to survive on so very little gruel. Hey, you win some, you lose some. So, unjust though it may be, we're going to work with your metabolism. That means eating fewer calories than you burn in order to lose weight, and you can do it.

If you're not eating much, but the weight isn't budging, you need to: 1) repair your brain so that it allows your metabolism to correct itself; and possibly 2) eat even less.

THIS IS SO &*#@ UNFAIR!

But, like so many American Indian tribes, a legacy of injustice is part of our history. Fighting what is, especially in our own genetic makeup, is a no-win proposition. Like Chief Joseph of the Nez Perce, all of us might want to reach the point where we say, "I will fight no more forever." Instead of being angry at our chubby genes, we can learn to be healthy by accepting our biological reality and adapting our way of life, like the Mexican Pima, so that we never have to be overweight.

FINDING JUSTICE IN 4 DAYS

The best way to tolerate the injustice is to remember what I heard, over and over, from people who had successfully lost a lot of weight and kept it off:

"I was only hungry for the first 4 days."
"I didn't notice it after 4 days."
"It was fine after the 4 days or so."
"The first 4 days were tough; after that, not bad."

This book is called *The 4-Day Win* because I want you to remember that you don't have to sustain a state of ravenous starvation for the rest of your life to be lean. In fact, that will inevitably make you fat. Just because you have a tendency to gain weight doesn't mean nature "wants you" to be extra large, any more than the Arizona Pima are "meant to" suffer from obesity and diabetes. If you're currently used to eating 10,000 calories a day, if you're using food as a calming drug, or have a naturally inefficient metabolism, losing weight will mean eating a lot less, and tolerating some hunger, sometimes. *But the sense of deprivation must be mild, never severe, and it should never last longer than 4 days.*

You're going to use 4-day wins, along with every single skill I've mentioned in this book, as you reduce your calorie intake enough to ensure you burn off extra weight, forever. Let's review a few of the main points, then get specific about how you, personally, are going to eat so much less that your excess body fat will become a distant memory.

- Learn to think of your body as a wary prey animal, a creature that doesn't respond well to force, anger, control, attack, sudden moves, or starvation. Learn to love your creature-self.
- Notice the difference between gut hunger and brain hunger. The first condition requires food. The second requires fixing a disordered craving pattern.
- Do not go to war on yourself or your appetite. Instead, access the part of your brain where only compassion and observation can occur—not fear, conflict, or compulsiveness. Become the Watcher any time you feel out of control, to structurally repair your brain.
- Habitually question all of your own thoughts that cause anxiety. Look for reasons they may not be true—because they aren't. Seeing that they are not true quiets the terrible stress created by your own mind, without making you eat.
- Become your own research project. Correlate events in your past with times when you became fatter or thinner, and notice which activities, people, and places in your present life cause you to feel like a rat in a trap.
- Get used to continually building a life that meets your real needs, desires, and destiny. By eliminating "rat trap" components and adding "rat park" elements, you'll create a life free from craving, including the craving for excess food.
- Experiment with different food combinations to see which foods satisfy you most while padding your rump the least. Focus on natural, unprocessed foods with simple flavors. Eat what you know your body wants.
- Make sure you have ample supplies of foods you love. Learn that food is abundant, that you will always have enough, that it's safe to discard leftovers because you live in a time and place of plenty.
- Make sure you aren't in a state of exhaustion (possible adrenal burnout). If you are, begin resting and relaxing more until you actually want to exert effort of some kind.
- Note your daily patterns of action (your daymap), and begin using your circadian rhythm to change the pattern each day, so that you end up in the right place to exercise more than you've done in the past. Repeat each new behavior on 4 consecutive days to establish your new daymap.

- Modify your daymap so that your body expects food only at the healthiest times.

There's just one skill set you have yet to learn—and you're about to learn it. In this chapter, we'll talk about: 1) reducing your eating to weight-loss levels without creating famine brain; 2) keeping your food at a level that ensures continued weight loss; and 3) *never getting fat again*. With all the skills you have, plus those you're about to learn, YOU CAN DO IT!

THE MOTHER OF ALL EXERCISES: BACKING OFF THE CHUCK WAGON

STEP 1: NOTICE HOW MUCH FOOD YOU TYPICALLY EAT DURING AN AVERAGE DAY

Start with your eating daymap, and possibly your food-mood-brood journal. Notice how much you typically eat. You'll need some way to make some rough calculation of your food intake. If you're on a diet you've found in a book or article, these sources will list the type and amount of food you're supposed to eat at each meal. If you're a calorie-counting type, go ahead and use calories as your measure. If you're on a program like Jenny Craig, the portions are already designed for you, and your counselor can help you adjust your food intake as you observe how your body reacts to the program. I've never met any weight-struggling person who didn't have some system of food-intake measurement. Use what works best for you.

STEP 2: REDUCE YOUR DAILY FOOD INTAKE BY ABOUT 100 CALORIES PER DAY

Again, your formal diet book or diet advisor can tell you how much food equals about 100 calories. You may decide to cut out the least healthy food on your menu, throw away a certain percentage of food at each meal, cut back on simple carbs like refined-flour bread, pie crust, and jawbreakers, or replace a very rich food with something that's less rich but still satisfying. *Don't cut out any of your favorite foods unless they are immediately lethal. Work on developing abundance brain by reminding yourself that you can always have these foods, just not to the point of feeling horribly stuffed, getting fat, and making yourself sick.*

PROPER ZONE FOR HUNGER DURING WEIGHT LOSS

Never let yourself get uncomfortably full or miserably hungry. As you reduce calories, 4 days at a time, you will feel more and more satisfied on less food with each 4-day win.

When your body is hungry, eat until satisfied. If your brain is hungry, or you can't eat enough to feel satisfied, use brain-calming strategies instead of food. This will take practice and experience, and *you won't to do it perfectly. That's okay. Just do it.*

0	1	2	3	4	5	6	7	8	9	10

Stuffed   Ideal Hunger Zone   Ravenous

Sustain this new level of food intake (about 100 calories a day less than you're used to) for 4 days. The entire time, stay in the middle of your "hunger range." If 0 equals stuffed to the gills, and 10 equals ravenous, you want to stay right in the middle. Ideally, don't let yourself get hungrier than a 6 or more full than a 4 (3 and 7 are acceptable, but risky). *Never let your hunger get above an 8; this creates famine brain.* It's better to slightly raise your intake to stay below an 8 on the hunger scale for this 4-day win. If you do this, you'll be able to handle eating less without hunger during your next 4-day win.

STEP 3: SUBSTITUTE INEDIBLE NOURISHERS (SIN) EVERY TIME YOU REDUCE YOUR FOOD INTAKE, AND AFTER EVERY MEAL OR SNACK

Don't make the mistake of trying to live some gulag lifestyle without either food or comfort. As you reduce calorie intake, increase the amount of time you spend feeding your soul. At the conclusion of every meal or snack, give yourself 5 to 15 minutes of nonfood pleasure, in any legal fashion you choose. Use relaxation and breathing exercises, "treasuring" visualizations, sights, smells, sounds, and memories that remind you of love and happiness.

Focus on your passions or hobbies, from spoon-hanging to shopping to learning about tectonic plate theory.

For 4-day win treats, indulge your inner Wild Child like a doting grandmother. SIN, SIN, SIN, to let your whole self know you're loved, catalyze the production of feel-good hormones, and give yourself infinite nonfood options for calming and delighting yourself at every level. This will help you tolerate the slight hunger you'll feel for 3 days. On the 4th day, you'll feel less physically hungry.

STEP 4: IF YOU'RE NOT LOSING WEIGHT, DROP YOUR FOOD INTAKE BY ABOUT ANOTHER 100 CALORIES PER DAY (AS CALCULATED BY YOU, YOUR DIETITIAN, A DIET BOOK, OR A WEIGHT-LOSS COUNSELOR)

As you keep lessening your food intake, you might feel a little hungry even if you're not losing weight yet. That's simply because your circadian rhythm is used to eating more than you actually need—and storing the extra food on your abundant pot belly. By reducing food gradually, adding nonfood nourishment, and giving your circadian rhythm 4 days to establish new expectations, you'll allow your body to stop wanting excessive food.

STEP 5: WATCH AND DEAL MENTALLY WITH ANY DEMONS THAT EMERGE INTO CONSCIOUSNESS, NOW THAT YOU'RE NOT USING FOOD AS A DRUG TO KEEP THEM REPRESSED

The mild hunger you may feel during the first 3 days of reduced food intake may scare you (actual hunger, however slight, is deeply unnerving to someone who has suffered repeated starvation). The fact that you aren't medicating your emotions with food may *terrify* you. All the demons you've been burying under baby-back ribs will emerge as you begin eating less and losing weight.

Bring out your food-mood-brood journal, and observe all sensations as well as thoughts. Watch any anxious mind-stories associated with the fear of future hunger, or of failing, or of succeeding, or that you'll be attacked by your deranged uncle, that no one has ever really loved you, that you have no talent, that your spouse is cheating, that your kids are going to disappear and never even visit you at the big-city bus station where you may spend your so-called "golden" years, even though you don't see anything golden about aging, which reminds you that you should bleach your teeth, because your high-school reunion is coming up and you're going to be the fat, yellow-toothed butt (BIG butt) of every joke, just like you were that time when in middle school when your physical education teacher yada yada yada yada *yada*.

In other words, the slight hunger you'll feel on the first 3 days of your 4-day win is a wonderful opportunity to examine your mind and address its dysfunctions, so that as you lose weight you'll become a happier and calmer person, not just a temporarily skinny food addict. Notice the stories that rise into your mind in the absence of food, go into the Watcher mode, and gently question each thought that causes anxiety. Are you certain your story is real, or is it just a tale told by an idiot, full of sound and fury, signifying nothing? No offense, but I think you'll find that the latter description fits reality better.

A final note on anxiety: *Remember that feeling frantic to lose 50 pounds by tomorrow is an anxious thought, and will keep you overweight.* Don't fight such thoughts, just observe them and offer yourself compassion. I'm not telling you this in order to force patience or to trap you in hell. I'm asking you to allay your own anxiety about rapid weight loss as well as everything else, because *this approach changes your brain into the brain of a skinny person.*

STEP 6: USE FLAVOR TRICKS TO LOWER YOUR HUNGER LEVEL (AND POSSIBLY YOUR FAT SET-POINT)

You'll feel a lot less hungry, and think about food less, if you use flavor tricks. Eat food with less intense or complex flavors—for example, real chicken instead of chicken that's been injected with sugar water, or oatmeal instead of a prepared oat cereal that's been engineered to increase your appetite by combining all sorts of flavors that you won't even notice—but which teach your brain to beg for more than you need.

As I said in Chapter 24, I've found that I can cut my appetite dramatically by using "flavor fasts," going an hour with no flavor of any kind, consuming a small amount of food that's high in calories but has no flavor (such a tasteless fish oil capsules) and then going another hour without flavors. This won't change any psychological hunger you might feel, but it may teach your brain to lower your hunger levels, and even your fat set point. Plus, most nutritionists highly recommend fish oil as a daily supplement; check with your doctor to make sure it's right for you.

STEP 7: KEEP CUTTING BACK ON FOOD, GRADUALLY, 4 DAYS AT A TIME, UNTIL YOU NOTICE A CHANGE IN YOUR BODY

If you continue edging your food intake down, you'll find that after a certain 4-day win (the one that takes you below the amount of food necessary to sustain your current weight) your body seems different. Even if you don't see much difference on your bathroom scale (yet), your clothes will be a little looser. You'll feel a little stronger, more mobile, more agile. The fat deposits on your body will begin losing fullness, like a balloon with the air leaking slowly away. This feeling, even more than the number on the scale (which may change due to water retention) is what tells you that you're losing weight.

STEP 8: LINK FIVE 4-DAY WINS TOGETHER TO MAKE WEIGHT LOSS COMPLETELY HABITUAL

Once you're 4 days into a weight-loss routine, the hard part is over. Maintain your eating at this level, and even though you'll keep losing weight, you won't feel like you're on some brutal, skin-of-your-teeth regimen. Losing weight will be normal, like walking your dog, talking to your children, driving to work, or washing the dishes—not completely free of effort, but so familiar and habitual that it certainly doesn't feel difficult. Once you've linked enough 4-day wins to add up to 21 days of dieting (five wins plus 1 day) research indicates that your new way of life will be a habit that's actually hard to break.

FINALLY: BE NICE TO YOURSELF

Once you're in the swing of your weight loss, feeling and seeing the fat disappear, knowing that you can keep losing weight without suffering, and exchanging your mental demons for Thinner Peace, you'll experience a steady rise in your optimism and sense of efficacy. This is the "early win" that development theorists have found results in permanent positive change. You are not becoming a skinny caterpillar—a thinner version of the old you. You're becoming a whole new animal, a gorgeous airy thing that will never return to caterpillar life.

To sustain this wonderful process, just remember not to fly too high, too fast. Get lots of rest. Never forget to give yourself the daily rewards, or the bigger rewards you "win" every 4 days. Keep your food intake level at a weight-loss level, but never let your body get ravenous. Never give in to the temptation to starve or overwork your body. If you're impatient, and find yourself wanting to starve or overwork yourself, return to the identity of the Watcher, observe your Dictator insisting on harmfully harsh tactics, and gently remind all parts of yourself that at any given moment, everything is okay.

Paradoxically, this loving acceptance of yourself, at every moment of your weight loss experience, is what fuels the process of metamorphosis. It's the way you clear a path to a slim, lean body no matter what genetic pattern you inherited from your ancestors, so that you'll naturally fight your own body no more, and eat a bit less, forever.

"I Will Eat a Bit Less Forever" 4-Day Win

Ridiculously Easy Daily Goal: *For the next 4 days, I'll slowly reduce the amount of food I eat, while increasing nonfood nourishment. I'll repeat this 4-day win until I reach a level that causes me to burn fat and drop pounds. I'll learn to recognize the feeling of "riding the edge" of hunger, and stay there while satisfying my emotional and physical need for non-food nourishment.*

Small Daily Reward: _____

_____

Slightly Larger 4-Day Reward: _____

_____

	Dates of My Current 4-Day Win	Check Off Completed Days Here
Day 1:	____ / ____ / ____	_____
Day 2:	____ / ____ / ____	_____
Day 3:	____ / ____ / ____	_____
Day 4:	____ / ____ / ____	_____

If you're already on a weight-loss regimen, remember that the 4-day win will enhance it, not conflict with it. If you know what to do, this program will help you do what you know. Feel free to stay on any weight-loss program while you learn 4-day win skills!

STAGE
5

MAINTENANCE

CHAPTER 33

TRIM-TABBING ALONG THE MIDDLE WAY

STAYING THIN
NO MATTER WHAT

T he Julias did not have time to stay thin. This was their consensus. They spoke about the problem in virtually identical terms, though none of them knew each other.

I met the Julias while writing this book: Three women, all with the same name (though it wasn't actually "Julia") asked me to help them understand why, after losing large amounts of weight, they'd been unable to maintain their hard-won slenderness. Julia #1 had lost more than 100 pounds, then regained 80. Julia #2 had lost 40, and bounced back up 50; when I met her, her weight was at an all-time high. And Julia #3 had lost, then gained, then lost, then gained, about 65 pounds.

When I called each Julia separately for get-to-know-you conversations, all three ascribed their most recent weight gain to stress and lack of time. "My job is a 24/7 proposition," said Julia #1, a hospital administrator, "and people depend on me. There just isn't a moment to focus on my own health."

"My parents are getting old, and they need a lot of help. On top of raising three kids, it's just been too much," said Julia #2.

"I'm juggling family and work," said Julia #3. "If I had any time and energy to stay fit, I would, but right now, everything and everyone else comes first."

Anyone who's ever taken on a tough job or family crisis can empathize with the Julias. I certainly do. But at the same time, their statements really didn't make sense. Like many Americans, the Julias manifested a tendency to think of maintaining a healthy weight as a big old time-gobbler. True, formal exercise takes time, but as we've seen, pacing around a room is a great calorie burner, and besides, moving more doesn't have nearly as much influence on weight as eating less. How much time and energy does it take to *not* eat an extra slice of cake? Does it take less time to munch a muffin than an apple? How is it that the less time we have, the more time we spend pigging out?

WILLPOWER WASTES WORK

Most people, including the Julias, never question the idea that staying thin takes huge amounts of time and energy. That's because almost all of us assume there's only one way to lose weight: by willpower, by white-knuckle resistance, by forcing the body with an aggressive, adversarial, disciplinarian mind. This can be achieved *sometimes,* though not often. Maintaining it long-term? I don't think that can be done.

All three Julias had shown incredible discipline, using their Dictator selves to trap, dominate, and starve their Wild Child selves. Losing weight this way is as draining as keeping a violent criminal pinned to the floor with sheer force. But even if you manage to do it, you can't hold your own Wild Child in a hammerlock for the rest of your life. The minute you get tired, distracted, or sick, the Dictator loses control, and the Wild Child goes into a feeding frenzy.

That's the whole reason I wrote this book. Simply going on a diet program, without changing your mental set, causes backlash and weight gain. *This is an inevitable reality, based on the way our brains and bodies are designed.* But if you use 4-day win techniques, your brain changes as well as your body. Weight loss happens without backlash or resistance, and as a result, maintaining it doesn't require time or energy. On the contrary, it allows you to relax, even under pressure.

I've lost weight the Julias' way several times, and just like them, I regained all the lost fat (and more) when I got busy, stressed, or tired. But since I started steering my brain to a place of compassionate observation and using 4-day wins, I've had much less difficulty maintaining the weight I prefer, no matter what. When I spent months too sick to get out of bed, let alone exercise, these techniques still worked. When I was on three different drugs that listed "weight gain" as a major side effect, they still worked. When I had three kids under 5, plus a doctoral program, plus a job, plus financial stress, they still worked. When my favorite contestant on *American Idol* was unfairly sent home—well, all right, I had a little relapse. But it was only temporary. I experienced plenty of pressures, but none of them resulted in significant weight gain.

That's why there's not a lot more for you to learn now that we've reached the maintenance stage of your 4-day win program. *If you practice and master the skills you've read about in earlier sections—especially the "Contemplation" stage—maintaining a healthy lifestyle and body weight will be virtually automatic.* Even better, these skills will give you more powerful, effective ways of coping with all your problems. You won't have to simply suffer without food as a comforter; instead, you'll find comfort without thinking about food. In fact, if you'll realize that life becomes less stressful as you learn to "not-think."

EXPLANATION: NOT-THINKING ALONG THE MIDDLE WAY

When I was a college student, obsessing about my weight as is customary for young American women in institutions of higher learning, I used to wonder why eating disorders were almost nonexistent in Asia. I majored in Chinese, and spent my junior year worrying about my weight all over Southeast Asia. The people there were all thin and gorgeous, and never seemed to think about their weight. I assumed this was a racial and dietary thing—these people were naturally skinny, and their food was slenderizing.

Unfortunately, no matter how much of that food I ate, it never slenderized me. My Singaporean friends, who collectively weighed less than either of my thighs, were always kidding me about laying off the chow mein. Never having worried about their weight for one single minute, my friends weren't at all tactful about mine. You would not believe how much chow mein it took to make me feel better.

More than 20 years later, according to journalistic reports, Asian girls and women are beginning to obsess about weight, just like Americans. Many analysts ascribe this to MTV and fast food. I disagree. I think the problem is Creeping Western Philosophy Syndrome. I think Asian culture has certain basic premises that are more conducive to Thinner Peace than the basic premises of Western thought. As Western culture spreads, so does fathead thinking and eating.

THE FATTENING "ISMS" OF WESTERN THOUGHT

The cultures that were born in the Middle East, and developed there and in Western Europe, focus on rationalism, domination, and being right. Judaism, Islam, and Christianity are all monotheistic religions. Each hold that there is one God, one way of being right, and we must all struggle toward it. Rationalism keeps this rigid thought structure in place, but replaces God with reason. "I think, therefore I am," said Descartes, and ever since, people in cultures where Western rationalism has taken root have equated their identities, their very existence, with their thoughts.

In many Asian philosophical traditions, on the other hand, the thinking self is called "monkey mind," and viewed as the resident idiot of the psychological village. "In the pursuit of knowledge," said Lao Tzu, "every day something is added. In the pursuit of enlightenment, every day something is dropped." The things Asian philosophers "dropped" on their way to enlightenment were delusions—thoughts that fuel neuroticism and overeating. Remember the permanently helpless Dalmatian reptile? Western thought encourages the very ways of seeing the world that Eastern philosophies gently disavow: the illusion of fixed states, learned helplessness, black-and-white thinking, and a worldview based on lack and attack.

The Julias, unknown to one another, had all gone deeper into these dysfunctional thought patterns when they lost weight. Their rational, force-based approach had deepened the famine response in their brains, intensified their cravings, made it ever harder to sustain the condition of willpower-based skinniness. They shared a mental state of extreme, perpetual anxiety. This was partly due to circumstances, but was much worse because of the way they'd dieted and regained weight, throughout their lives. The Julias had starved and abused their bodies, all the time thinking this was somehow righteous, so their bodies were trying desperately to get fatter.

So we began changing the way the Julias thought. They all learned and practiced contemplation exercises to soothe their panic and send the energy of their brains away from compulsivity, into the energy of the Watcher. Within one day, all three women told me their eating felt less compulsive. Instead of thinking their way thin, they'd begun learning the contemplative's skill of not-thinking. Immediately, the psychological pressure to gain weight decreased, and their ability to cope calmly with their busy, stressful lives increased. They were on the way to healing the "craving brain" syndrome that had been so exacerbated by the way they'd dieted in the past—and as their brains change, their bodies are getting thinner.

THE MIDDLE WAY

Another theme that's stronger in Asian thought than in the West is simply moderation. Ancient Western images of "perfect" humans are extreme: they seek poverty, starve themselves, whip themselves, whip other people. The Buddha, archetypal role model of Asia, wasn't into that. You might think so if you saw only the statues that portray Siddhartha as a fat happy camper, beaming over a beer gut the size of a Subaru or the other Buddha images that have washboard ribs and sunken (though serene) eyes. Buddhist tradition says that after covering all the bases in extreme living, as one scholar puts it,

> . . . later the Buddha rejected extreme asceticism as an impediment to ultimate freedom from suffering, choosing instead a path that met the needs of the body without crossing over into luxury and indulgence. *After abandoning extreme asceticism he was able to achieve enlightenment.* [italics added]

Enlightenment in the West is all about self-deprivation. In Eastern thought, it's about choosing the Middle Way of lovingly detached self-acceptance. Returning over and over to this mental position, as do the Tibetan monks, whose brains show unusual levels of health, is the single most important thing you can do to stay slender once you've lost your extra weight. This doesn't mean you won't have to think about eating right and staying active. You'll just become more and more able to think about them with high levels of efficacy, and low levels of stress.

EXERCISE: MAKING TRIM TAB ADJUSTMENTS

Remember trim tabs, those little mini-rudders that make big rudders functional? Don't ever forget that 4-day wins are weight-control trim tabs you can use forever.

If you've lost weight and then begin to regain, you simply alter your behavior for 4 days to get back on course. This works no matter how much weight you've regained, and if you make "trim tab" adjustments as part of everyday living, you'll never be more than 4 days away from your ideal weight.

I'm about to suggest something that is discouraged by most diet counselors. But research on maintaining slenderness after weight loss shows that it's very effective. It is . . . read the whole chapter before you react . . . weighing yourself on a daily basis. You are hearing this from someone who, on multiple occasions, refused to seek medical attention after being seriously wounded, for fear the doctor would weigh me. To those of us who have experienced the horrors of yo-yo dieting, the scale is more alarming than the rack, the lash, and thumbscrews combined.

But weighing in is traumatic only when we have anxious thoughts about the whole process. Even though I was leery of weighing myself during my binge-and-starve days, I now do it every day without anxiety, even when I've gained weight. When I begin feeling anxious, I go straight to my Watcher mental position. I examine my panicky thoughts ("Oh no! I'm blimping up like a puffer fish!") and question them. From the Watcher's observational standpoint, I no longer feel the anxiety. I steer myself toward eating a bit less and moving a bit more without becoming the abusive Dictator. According to researchers from the Centers for Disease Control and Prevention, daily weigh ins were highly correlated with sustaining weight loss. If it works for me, it'll work for anybody.

USING THE SCALE AS A TRIM-TAB NAVIGATOR, NOT A TORTURE DEVICE

To keep your 4-day wins in the "trim tab" range, rather than veering way off course and trying to turn so abruptly that you rupture something, I strongly recommend getting a good scale and weighing in practically every morning.

When I say "practically," it's because I allow myself one exception: On the day after I've had an extremely intense, A-level workout, I don't weigh myself. Why? Because tearing down muscle tissue, which is what you do in hard training, makes the muscle tissue retain water in order to repair itself. This is why weight-lifters "get pumped" by working out hard right before a competition—the extra water drawn into the muscle actually makes it bigger. It's also heavier, though the extra weight is fluid, not fat or muscle.

One of the things that discourages my clients most is that they work out like crazy right before the a weigh in, trying to drop the pounds—which means they actually weigh more when they climb on the scale. Wrestlers, jockeys, and other athletes who have to "make weight" avoid this problem by combining heavy workouts with dehydration. They sweat as much as they can, without drinking any water. This will indeed make you weight less. So will hacking off one of your limbs. Dehydration is very bad for you. People die from it. Short recommendation: Don't. Long recommendation: I'm serious. Don't.

STEERING BACK TO THINNER PEACE

The skills you've been picking up as you've read through this book are all you need to tweak the trim tabs on your diet and exercise, steering you back to the weight you want. But remember, this won't just change the amount you eat and move. It will change your whole life. Remember Rat Park. If your weight begins to climb, and you observe yourself as the compassionate Watcher, you may find that some aspect of your life situation is causing some sort of unhappiness that motivates overeating. Just being serene won't always be enough to put you back in the zone where you don't need to self-medicate with food.

From the Watcher perspective, you can see when weight gain is related to stressors in your family life, your career, your friendships, your health, the way the White House is dealing with issues that matter to you, etc. Then you can choose to respond in a way that addresses the actual problem—again, using trim tab actions, not massive disruptions. You'll have a much more positive impact on your loved ones, your job prospects, and international politics (and everything in between) if you don't react to them solely by inhaling pans of blueberry cobbler.

It didn't take long for the Julias to start making trim-tab changes in their lives, not just their bodies, once they began using 4-day win techniques. Julia #1 is still a hospital administrator, but she's now "bagged, bettered, and bartered" some of her work tasks, takes daily 30-minute "meditation walks" that have reduced her stress, feels back in control of her eating, and has lost about 30 pounds. Julia #2 began using 4-day win psychological strategies while caring for her father after he had a stroke. She found that it not only calmed her, allowing her to eat less, but seemed to have a positive effect on her dad. And Julia #3 has begun caring for herself as well as her kids and her job, with daily 15-minute "meditation workouts" to address adrenal-burnout-level exhaustion. She, too, has stopped compulsive eating.

All these women are as busy as humanly possible. But when it comes to maintaining weight with the constant gentle application of 4-day win techniques, they're less tired, not more. Losing the weight they've regained is healing their brains, not damaging them further. And all of them, contrary to everything they'd ever experienced before, have found that when it comes to maintaining a healthy weight, there's always plenty of time.

"Trim Tab Adjustment" 4-Day Win

Ridiculously Easy Daily Goal: *For the next 4 days, I'll weigh myself every morning (except the morning after an A-level workout). If I've gained weight, I won't freak out; instead, I'll go to the place of Thinner Peace and make small, trim-tab changes in my eating and exercise patterns to correct course and drop extra fat before it's a major issue.* _____

Small Daily Reward: _____

_____

Slightly Larger 4-Day Reward: _____

_____

	Dates of My Current 4-Day Win	Check Off Completed Days Here
Day 1:	____ / ____ / ____	_____
Day 2:	____ / ____ / ____	_____
Day 3:	____ / ____ / ____	_____
Day 4:	____ / ____ / ____	_____

If you're already on a weight-loss regimen, remember that the 4-day win will enhance it, not conflict with it. If you know what to do, this program will help you do what you know. Feel free to stay on any weight-loss program while you learn 4-day win skills!

STAGE
6

RELAPSE

CHAPTER 34

GETTING BACK ON THE HORSE

RELAPSE AND RECOVERY

Nute is what horse people call a "trail-broke gelding." He's huge—part draft horse—but fairly mellow, used to being ridden by visitors to the mountain resort where he lives. Unless he feels really, really threatened, Nute is a well-behaved, compliant horse. Which makes it seems strange that I am deliberately making him feel really, really threatened.

"Horses are terrified of plastic bags," my horse-whisperer friend Koelle Simpson just informed me. Then she gave me a short stick with several plastic bags attached to one end and told me to go up to Nute and shake the bags at him. She might as well have said, "Hey, dude, eat this, it's totally poisonous!"

But because I'm human, and thus have far less sense than your average horse, I followed Koelle's instructions. Now I'm rushing around in the circular pen waving Nute's worst nightmare in his face, staying as close as I can to this enormous beast as he shies away, tries to bolt, rolls his eyes, sweats, and generally freaks out. We rush around like this until Nute gets a little tired and starts to relax. Then, still following Koelle's directions, I move the bags away. Nute stops shaking quite as hard.

"Again," says Koelle, perhaps annoyed that Nute hasn't killed me yet.

I push the bags at Nute again, and he tries to bolt again, but this time he gets a little calmer a little sooner. I pull the bags away.

After several iterations, Nute doesn't seem nearly as frightened. He's begun to realize something counterintuitive: getting scared and running away from the bags makes them follow him everywhere, while relaxing and ignoring them makes them go away. Many traditionally "broken" horses never overcome their violent fear of plastic bags. But within about 5 minutes, Nute is no longer bag-phobic. He just stands there politely, flicking his tail every now and again, as I shake the bags in his face, brush them against his body, snap them in the air next to his ears.

"Once the horse trusts you," Koelle says, "we actually want to bring up fear and anxiety, so that we can teach him that there's less and less in the world he needs to be afraid of. He's also learning to accept you as his leader. He'll be more and more cooperative with you as his fear goes down and his trust in you goes up."

RELAPSE MEANS "RELAX!"

Once again, horse whispering amazes me with its similarity to weight management. In Chapter 5, we talked about how typical diets put you in direct opposition to your body's instincts, the way a predator is at odds with a prey animal. Losing weight without causing "famine brain" requires body whispering from the very beginning. The aspect of horse training I'm learning with Nute has everything in common with how to handle weight-related relapses.

"Relapse" is the sixth stage in the transtheoretical model of change. Everyone goes through it. Eating is just so ubiquitous, "bad" food so plentiful, and life so stressful that no one can be a perfectly healthy eater all the time. Or at least, no one you and I would want in our immediate circle.

Willpower-based weight losers, with their black-and-white thought patterns, often give up entirely when they relapse. My friends at Jenny Craig told me many stories of successful dieters who decided to throw in the towel after a single slip-up. "What we're trying to teach clients," said Lisa Talamini, head of product development, "is that relapses are actually opportunities to build more trust in your program and your body."

Sound familiar? It probably would to Nute.

So if you're relapsing—if this chapter has caught you elbow-deep in a trough of mashed potatoes—please be assured that you haven't made a terrible mistake. You've just given yourself a lovely opportunity to gain even more confidence that you can stay thin for life.

EXPLANATION: YOUR BODY'S HORSE SENSE

If you've done the exercises designed to facilitate peaceful coexistence between your mind and body, they should be getting much more comfortable with one another. In a best-case scenario, they've become affectionate allies. Your body tells you what it needs (lots of kindness, yummy food, bounteous supplies, no outright starvation). By the same token, your mind lets your body know what it wants (eat a bit less, exercise a bit more, get healthier and look better in tight jeans). You listen to your body and respect its wishes, so it returns the favor. The two of you are a happy team, just like the Lone Ranger and Silver.

Then one day, you're riding along on the range, and Silver goes batcrap crazy—bucking, rearing, trying to bite you. In other words, your body stops following directions and goes back to old dysfunctional eating patterns. One minute your weight-control program is going fine, and the next, you're polishing off an entire pie. Or perhaps it happens slowly; just when you're confident that your body is always going to sustain healthy habits, you realize that your weight has crept up, that you're eating more and enjoying it less, that the most challenging exercise you undertake is raising your arm to signal the waiter at the Crouch 'n' Crunch BBQ Buffet. Silver (that's your body, if you're tracking the metaphor) has wandered off the path of healthy living and is taking you right back to the dreaded, desolate Fatlands.

UH-OH, SILVER

So how do you handle a relapse? By giving up? Many people do this, and go through months of weight gain until they hate themselves enough to starve again. Not a good idea. Do you crack down on your body, decide that you could never trust that no-good animal anyway, and start ruling it with control tactics? This, too, will lead to the nightmare of oscillating fatness that has already blighted too much of your life.

No, when you relapse into overeating or under-exercising, and your weight is going back up, the best advice is to take your body-whispering skills to the next level. Stay with your body in its panic. Tolerate your own fear and confusion. Stay as present as possible, even in your bingeing. Follow the instructions in Chapter 10, thinking through your "misbehavior" and

paying attention to your feelings. Above all, refuse to hate or condemn yourself. If Silver got a bit too frisky, do you think the Lone Ranger would shoot
him? Of course not! He'd make Tonto do it! (But Tonto wouldn't, because
Tonto was always a lot sharper than the Lone Ranger—I mean, what was he
hiding with that ridiculous mask? Acne?)

Seriously, if Silver acted up, the Lone Ranger would pay attention,
because he'd know that one of three things was true: 1) Silver was hurt or
scared for some legitimate reason; 2) Silver had spotted a plastic bag, or
other object he didn't understand; or 3) Silver knew that the Lone Ranger
was headed in the wrong direction, and he was trying to get L.R. to wake up
and smell the buffalo chips.

Weight-gain or bingeing relapse is your body freaking out for the same
reasons Silver might. Relapse is your body's signal that something is wrong.
You don't know it consciously, because *you've relegated some issue to the pre-
contemplation part of your mind—in other words, gone into denial.* You
wouldn't be relapsing if you weren't in denial about something. The knowledge you're hiding from yourself could be mild, or quite dramatic. But you
must face it if you want to be healthily thin for the rest of your life. Your job
(that is, the job of your thinking mind) is to stop, relax, and pay attention
until you realize what your body is trying to say.

EXERCISE: GETTING BACK
ON THE HORSE

A relapsing body is trying to tell its owner one or more of the same three
things Silver might be telling his rider. Each possibility requires a different
course of action, which will be your "exercise" should you find yourself getting a little too free with the cupcakes.

POSSIBILITY ONE: SOMETHING MAY BE WRONG
WITH YOUR BODY

Gabrielle has a tendency to get caught up in the excitement of her high-
pressure job and ignore her own physical fatigue. She goes into denial about
the fact that she's really tired and needs to sleep a little more. If she doesn't
accept this truth and give her body more rest, she gains weight.

For Cynthia, weight gain signaled a more serious problem. A friend
recommended some herbal treatments for hot flashes. Cynthia took them

without a second thought. She began gaining weight hand over fist and felt constantly exhausted. She blamed menopause. Her doctor tried all sorts of fixes, but none of them worked—until Cynthia finally mentioned the herbal supplements to her doctor. Though the herbs work well for most people, it turned out Cynthia was allergic to them, and that allergy was creating fatigue, systemic inflammation, and weight gain.

SOLUTION: PAY CLOSE ATTENTION TO YOUR BODY, AND GET PROFESSIONALS TO HELP

If you sense there's something wrong, don't give up on yourself even if the first person you consult can't help. I spent 12 years in constant pain until a friend kept pushing me to new specialists, one of whom finally gave me the right diagnosis and treatment.

POSSIBILITY TWO: YOUR CREATURE-SELF IS SCARED OF SOMETHING THAT ISN'T REALLY DANGEROUS

In Chapter 12, I explained how anxiety levels go up when we have frightening thoughts. In fact, most of our anxiety is in response to thoughts, not our actual situation. I've watched hundreds and hundreds of clients sit in safe, warm, comfortable rooms and shake with terror about things that had never happened, and would never happen.

"I'll run out of money! I'll be a bag lady!"
"I'll be alone forever! No one ever loved me, and no one ever will!"
"Everyone's gossiping about me! And it will get even worse!"
"If I ever slip up, the captain of my curling team will get rid of me!"

Fears like these affect us just like plastic bags affect horses: we're terrified of them because we don't realize they're harmless. *They are only thoughts.* Sure, bad things happen to people. Some have happened to you before, and others will happen in the future. And, as I've said before, you'll live through all but one. The point is, once you've taken all legitimate precautions to avoid likely dangers, it's dysfunctional to continue to experience escalating anxiety, anger, or grief because you're so busy telling yourself about events that exist only in your mind.

Betty started gaining weight after September 11, 2001. She lives in New Jersey and travels by air a lot, and the World Trade Center attacks put her into a tailspin of fear even more severe than most of us experienced. Every time she had to fly, Betty would binge on cheap, nasty junk food. Her doctor put her on tranquilizers, which helped a little, but also made Betty's body more inclined to gain weight. This added self-loathing to Betty's daily mental story, along with the fear that her husband wouldn't be attracted to her unless she stayed skinny—which, of course, made her eat like the Apocalypse was upon her.

It took every sane person a long, long time to come to terms with 9/11; in some ways, none of us ever will. But Betty's constant panic wasn't making her any safer from terrorists. Instead, it led to a vicious cycle of increasingly paranoid fictions, of which weight gain was just one symptom. But that's the thing about red-blooded American women: they will do almost anything to lose weight. So, with a therapist's help, Betty began observing, analyzing, and questioning her own thoughts. She came to see the difference between a frightening reality and a frightening thought, and she realized that the latter, though genuinely unnerving, could not hurt her. *A scary thought has no power to hurt you unless you believe it.*

SOLUTION: USE YOUR WATCHER PERSPECTIVE
TO QUESTION ALL YOUR SCARY THOUGHTS

By going to the mental position of the Watcher, you can begin examining your own scary thoughts and seeing through them. They may well be full of sound and fury, but they signify nothing. When you see that, they will eventually go away, and certainly lose their power to cause overeating.

POSSIBILITY THREE: YOUR MIND IS TAKING
YOUR LIFE IN THE WRONG DIRECTION

When Barry lost control of his eating and gained 50 pounds in 2 years, it was because he knew in his heart that his marriage was over. Barry couldn't handle *really knowing* what he really knew, and as his relationship with his wife grew frailer, balanced precariously atop the lie that "everything's fine," Barry found himself overeating more and more severely. The day he finally decided to file for divorce, his bingeing stopped. Though the following years were very difficult, Barry never went back to pretending everything was fine. He courageously experienced all the tumultuous emotions appertaining to divorce, got support from friends and family, and lost weight even as he grieved.

I have always believed that my clients know in their hearts what their lives are meant to be. I've also found, in dealing with hundreds of people, that the body tends to stay more faithful to this inner knowing than the mind. In Asia they say, "The mind is a wonderful servant, but a terrible master." When a person's body is somehow "misbehaving," it's often because he or she is consciously trying to do something he or she unconsciously knows is wrong. I wrote a whole book about what to do in these cases (it's called *Finding Your Own North Star,* if you're interested) but all the knowledge you need is coded into your true self. All your 4-day win skills are meant to help you tune into that self. Once you realize what it's telling you, you have two choices: follow your destiny, or (if you're an overeater) get fat.

SOLUTION: CHANGE THE DIRECTION OF YOUR LIFE TO ACCORD WITH YOUR HEART'S DESIRES

This is rarely easy, and I myself would never try it without backup. A therapist can help if your loved ones aren't helpful, or you can hire a life coach like me to cheer you on as you forge a new, true future.

Joseph Campbell wrote, "You must give up the life you had planned in order to have the life that is waiting for you." As you realize how much happier your true life will be than the one you had planned, you'll be ever so grateful that your body pushed you to change, even if that meant putting on a temporary double chin.

GETTING BACK IN THE SADDLE

So, what's Silver trying to tell you, Kemosabe? Are you burned out, fed up, all in? Are you hiding things from yourself that you absolutely need to know? Whatever those things are, you'll find that relapses alert you to their presence. If you stay calm and stay with your 4-day win program, the problem will go away. If you go back into force-based thinking, relapse will follow you everywhere. It's all good, as long as you remember that "relapse" means "relax!"

Which is exactly what Nute and I finally do, together.

"See?" said Koelle, as I rub Nute's massive flank with the plastic bags and he lets out a contented sigh. "Every time you confront something scary together, you trust each other more. Bringing up a problem is just a chance to become a better team."

It's clear she's right. I suddenly adore this big guy, and he's nuzzling me gently, as if I'm the human he's been looking for all his life. The next time I have a relapse and my body starts lunging for munchies, I'll see it as an opportunity, not a curse. I'll make it work for my health and sanity, not against them. So hiyo, Nute, away!

"Back in the Saddle" 4-Day Win

Ridiculously Easy Daily Goal: *For the next 4 days, I'll go to my place of*

Thinner Peace and try to figure out what my relapse is trying to tell me about

my life. _____

Small Daily Reward: _____

_____

Slightly Larger 4-Day Reward: _____

_____

	Dates of My Current 4-day Win	Check Off Completed Days Here
Day 1:	_____ / _____ / _____	_____
Day 2:	_____ / _____ / _____	_____
Day 3:	_____ / _____ / _____	_____
Day 4:	_____ / _____ / _____	_____

If you're already on a weight-loss regimen, remember that the 4-day win will enhance it, not conflict with it. If you know what to do, this program will help you do what you know. Feel free to stay on any weight-loss program while you learn 4-day win skills!

STAGE
7

CELEBRATION

CHAPTER 35

DETERMINATION YIELDS DE TERMINATION

CELEBRATING FREEDOM

O ne of the darkest memories of my life is of a time when I should have felt all bright and shiny. I was sitting in a huge theater with a group of friends, listening to some awesome musicians deliver a great performance. I was young, relatively successful, surrounded by people who loved me, living in a state of abundance far beyond the dreams of the vast majority of humans beings who ever existed. Unfortunately, I wasn't actually experiencing any of it.

Loud as the music was, my brain barely registered it amid the chaos of my thoughts—the kind of thoughts that, for thousands of years, drove my caveman ancestors to focus so entirely on digging up edible roots that they rarely if ever took time to attend a concert.

I'd been living in diet hell for so long I might as well have spent my own life in a cave. All I could think about was food and weight, weight and food. How much had I eaten that day? What should I eat later? How could I keep myself from bingeing that night, as I'd binged every night for weeks? Why did I want to eat, even though I hadn't been hungry for a long time? Surges of panic flooded me every time I shifted in my chair and felt the tightness of my clothing. I was wearing my "fat" clothes, but even they had become too small. At an intellectual level, I knew it was stupid to be nearly insane with fear and self-hatred just because a roll of fat was bulging over the waistband of my jeans, but I couldn't quiet the hurricane in my head.

I remember staring at the musicians and trying desperately to just watch and listen, to stop obsessing about food and body size, to simply enjoy what was happening around me. I couldn't. I couldn't even remember what it was like to have any mental experience different from my own. I glanced at the skinny guy next to me and wondered what he thought about; I couldn't imagine what might fill a human mind if weight and food obsessions didn't.

At that time, I didn't understand the mechanisms in my own brain and body that brought me to such a sorry pass. I didn't know that my repeated dieting had changed the architecture of my brain, turning it into a food-obsessed, weight-gaining machine. I didn't know this was the inevitable result of the weight-management methods being touted by almost every expert in my culture. I was only sure that I hadn't known peace for as long as I could remember.

THAT WAS THEN, THIS IS NOW

Flash forward to the present day. I've reached an age (the Late Bronze Age) where most of my Baby Boomer peers—even the skinny guy I sat next to at that concert—are struggling to control their weight. I've just finished cruising the aisles at my local supermarket, picking up my favorite foods, which are (seriously) nuts and berries. True, I'm also buying a very large box of cookies. I may eat one or two of them, but mainly I'll *have* them, which will satisfy the ghost of famine-brain that's still in my head. Though most of the cookies will go stale and end up in my backyard bird feeder, I'm buying peace for my hording brain. It's well worth the few dollars I'm "wasting."

I notice absent-mindedly that the woman in front of me in the "10 items or less" line is purchasing, at a conservative estimate, 3,574 items. She also seems to be insisting that she wants to pay in an unorthodox fashion, say in expired coupons, loose pennies, and a small flock of grazing animals. So I've been standing in line for approximately an academic year, glancing over the magazines next to the counter. What I see is an echo of the time I spent trapped in my own binge-and-starve Torment of the Damned. The cover lines shout:

- Department of Health and Human Resources Announces 64 Percent of Americans Overweight or Obese!
- Bake a Cake NO ONE Can Pass Up! Recipe Inside!
- Ten Celebrities Who've Gotten Dangerously Fat! Pics on Page 15!
- Conquer Cellulite And Be 10 Pounds Thinner In 6 Weeks!
- Your Whole Family Will Want Seconds Of This 5-Cheese Casserole!

- Celebrities Wasting Away From Excessive Dieting—See Page 145!
- Blast Your Abs And Flatten That Tummy Now!
- Alien with Tom Cruise's DNA Marries Angelina Jolie, Produces Off-spring So Beautiful, Yet Somehow Disturbing, that Entire World Converts to Scientology In Attempt to Placate It!

So it's not just me. Our whole society has fallen victim to weight obsession. We overeat and starve, overeat and starve, pushing our brain structures further and further into a preoccupation with fat and food and programming ourselves to crave a blizzard of edibles unlike anything ever seen by any other species, at any other time in history. We have become a people of insane contradictions, demanding bigger portions while desperately trying to eat less, fighting like pit bulls for a parking space 50 feet closer to the gym, so that we don't have to walk to the place where we pay hundreds of dollars to exercise.

All because of the odd confluence of ancient biology and recent advances that have given us more food, and saved us more labor, than nature ever anticipated. The social and medical pressure to stay thin, combined with all this abundance, is making millions of people feel just as crazy as I did that long-ago night at the concert.

The program I've outlined in this book will empower you to negotiate this thicket of contradictions without losing yourself. I've benefited from every 4-day win in this program, and seen many of my clients benefit as well. By the time you've internalized all these practices, you too can come home to your body, trust your appetite, and become a thin, healthy person in the midst of the "obesity crisis."

EXPLANATION: NO TERMINATION, JUST CELEBRATION

The final stage of the transtheoretical model of change, as authors Prochaska and DiClemente labeled it, is "Termination." To a researcher studying bad habits in general, this means that a person no longer smokes any tobacco, does drugs, steals small objects from department stores, or blends and guzzles piña coladas in the office supply closet.

I'm not going to use the word "Termination" to describe the completion of the 4-day win, for two reasons. For one thing, eating is something you never "terminate," until you really have very little else on your appointment calendar ("9 a.m. Wednesday, rendezvous with Death; cancel lunch at Four Seasons"). That takes me to the second thing: "Termination" sounds like kicking the bucket, or at the very least being fired from a job. That's not what it feels like to love living in your own skin. That's not what it feels like at all. Instead of termination, it's celebration.

Nothing about me, body or mind, will ever be perfect. But I no longer need it to be. It's enough that I've regained the freedom to be present in my imperfect life. Having once lost my ability to experience life as anything but a grueling fitness project, I now experience even the most ordinary moments as extraordinarily delicious.

I also feel little inclination to eat unless I'm truly, physically hungry, so I haven't had to worry about my weight for a long time. The biggest problem I have when it comes to helping clients lose weight is that once they meet me, they assume I have no idea what it's like to be fat (when we meet over the phone, and they aren't biased by visual images, they sense immediately that I can empathize with them).

I still experience a ghostly vestige of my old, chubbier mindset when I'm under stress or scrutiny. It still makes me want to binge, still haunts me with the fear that I'll expand like a puffer fish any minute now. But the fear, self-hatred, and inclination to pig out don't last more than a few minutes, because now I know what to do about them. Every time I feel myself tense up, every time I criticize my own flesh or wince at the sight of the doctor's scale, I simply return to the perspective of the Watcher, the part of my awareness that observes everything, including my own thoughts, with compassion. The longer I continue to do this, the more I may be changing the structure of my brain, so that my old starve-and-binge dysfunction grows weaker, the capacity for appreciation stronger.

It's such a gentle process, this change. It's nothing like the aggressive, force-based strategies offered in every magazine at the supermarket. "The Way nourishes by not forcing," said Lao Tzu, and whenever I remember not to force, I find myself nourished in ways I never expected. I know you can be nourished in these ways, too.

EXERCISE: CELEBRATION

Faith, hope, and love, says the Good Book, are the most powerful tools a human being has to work with. For your first 4-day win, many eons ago, I asked you to open yourself up to hope. If you've done the work in the chapters between that one and this one, you will by now have experienced at least brief moments of love—not the grasping, possessive, or controlling need that sometimes passes for love, but absolute acceptance, without any need at all. This is the essence of the compassionate Watcher within you, who can extend genuine kindness to your most condemnatory Dictator aspects, and your most rebellious Wild Child side.

For this exercise, I want you to offer yourself not only basic good wishes ("May you be well, may you be happy, may you be free from suffering"), but congratulations and pride in your achievements. I want you to celebrate everything you've done that's brought you to this point in your life. Just by reading this book, you've begun freeing your brain from the constant vacillation between dieting and overeating. If you have learned to feel even the slightest bit of unconditional love for yourself, your weight history, and your body, you have begun a profound self-transformation that, if sustained, will inevitably continue to improve your physical and mental health. That deserves some celebration. So, then:

Party of One

1. Get a bottle or glass of the purest, iciest, clearest water you can find.

You can substitute some other beverage, if you like; juice or green tea or something, as long as it's good for you. Anything without high-fructose corn syrup, which, as previously noted, is devil-sweat and will kill you as soon as you look at it.

2. Find a quiet spot where you can sit for at least 10 minutes without interruption.

Take your beverage with you, as well as this book, your food-mood-brood journal, and any other journal or record where you've written about your own experience.

3. Consider your history.

Think about this for a minute: You are the product of countless beings who beat the odds by surviving long enough to reproduce, while countless others did not. Think of all the perils that beset your ancestors, for thousands and thousands of years. Your very existence is an almost incomprehensible miracle, and a gift from these generations of forebears. It was their survival advantage that helped them live when others starved. Drink to your ancestors. Cheers!

4. Consider the time in which you live.

For the last few millennia, your species has been developing such under-standing of natural law that we have now created wealth and plenty beyond anything this planet has ever seen. At the very same time human brains have been pushing forward toward mastery over nature, the wise men and women of all cultures, the great spiritual leaders from all traditions, have been exper-imenting to find ways in which the astonishing human brain can be kept from causing harm. You live at a time when these two great rivers of thought are converging, when science is able to watch the brain change as a result of deep contemplation, and when contemplatives can see scientific evidence of the way their strategies actually work.

This is an astonishing time to be human. Drink to it. Cheers!

5. Consider all you have overcome.

No one reading this book is unacquainted with sorrow. If you've been fat in a culture that simultaneously feeds you and mocks you; if you've endured shame, insecurity, and fear with dignity; if you've tried and failed and tried and failed and still pulled yourself together to try again; if you've endured starvation, weight obsession, the mind and heart-wounds inflicted by your attempts to somehow "do better"; if you've ever done any of these things, you've shown courage at a very high level, probably without giving yourself credit. And you're still here. Drink to that. Cheers!

6. Consider all you have achieved.

You probably spend far more time thinking about your failings than your successes, and right now, for the next few minutes, I want that to change. List 10 good things you have done in your life. Now 10 more. And 10 more. Remember times when you have done good when it was possible to do evil, when you've refrained from inflicting harm, when you've offered kindness and comfort. Recall 10 times you did things right. Ten times you learned from a mistake. Ten times other people have told you that you've made their lives better. You're really quite an amazing person, aren't you? Drink to that, and then drink to it again. Cheers! Cheers! Cheers!

AND FINALLY, FAITH

The saying "charity never faileth" rings true to me; because no matter what's going on in your life, you can choose to take a compassionate view of the forces that made you what you are. Now that you've exercised hope and love, I'd like you to do a little tango with faith. Just for a moment, stop trying to make your body fit some external standard, and—just for a moment, I said—*let go of all disbelief* in yourself, your body, your success losing weight, your future. You can go back to worrying and hating yourself as soon as this celebration is over, though I hope you'll choose to return to faith many, many times to come.

If you can willingly suspend disbelief that your 4-day win program will work—is working—you'll find that you forget to be obsessed or self-conscious for that time. Accept your body as it is right now, not to make yourself stay fat, but in the interests of a skinnier you, and then see how your body accepts this moment. You may experience a sense of the celebration that can become your continuous condition as you grow more and more practiced at your 4-day win skill. Suddenly, life won't be about fat any more. It will be about living.

This, your body will tell you—this line of type, this pool of light, this loved one's touch, this smell of rain, this sorrow or gladness, whatever this exists for you at this moment—this, this, this is your life. The fulfillment you think will come with winning the weight war is available to you right now, the moment you step back from the battlefield. That's the only skill you need to become the person you were meant to be, physically and in every other way. As my favorite philosophy dude Lao Tzu said,

> She who is centered in the way
> can go where she wishes, without danger.
> She perceives the universal harmony,
> even amid great pain,
> because she has found peace in her heart.

So there is no "termination" in your 4-day win program, only celebration. As long as you've got 4 days left, you can link those days into a gradually rising path to healthy, relaxed, skinny living. You'll find *de*termination there, to be sure. Also fitness, confidence, rapture, fulfillment, vibrancy, and joy. And, even at the times when life gets difficult (as it inevitably does) you will sense that beneath all these sparkling delights you have lit within your self a steady, calm, unquenchable flame of peace.

Thinner peace.

"Celebration" 4-Day Win

Ridiculously Easy Daily Goal: _For the next 4 days, I will take time to accept myself, my body, and my life as they are, and celebrate the progress I've made in self-understanding, recovery from the wounds of weight obsession, and experiencing Thinner Peace._

Small Daily Reward: _____

_____

Slightly Larger 4-Day Reward: _____

_____

	Dates of My Current 4-Day Win	**Check Off Completed Days Here**
Day 1:	____ / ____ / ____	_____
Day 2:	____ / ____ / ____	_____
Day 3:	____ / ____ / ____	_____
Day 4:	____ / ____ / ____	_____

If you're already on a weight-loss regimen, remember that the 4-day win will enhance it, not conflict with it. If you know what to do, this program will help you do what you know. Feel free to stay on any weight-loss program while you learn 4-day win skills!

APPENDIX

THE 4-DAY WIN JUMP-START
WEIGHT-LOSS PROGRAM

On the following pages you'll find a reprint of Chapters 6, 10, 21, and 32, clumped together for your reading convenience, into a 4-day win weight loss program. You can always read them the context of the larger program, and they'll make sense in more ways, on more levels, as you get more context by reading the rest of the book. You'll only change your brain into a lean machine, as opposed to a fat-conservationist, by integrating the concepts and skills in the other chapters.

But to get you started on your physical transformation, and to give you that first, crucial 4-day win where you see and feel changes in your body, read through these chapters as a group, and implement the suggestions they contain. Once you're on the weight-loss program, you can read, master, and integrate your brain-changing "thinner peace" skills as you continue to lose weight. You'll find your weight loss feeling more natural, and you'll have fewer problems with rebounding, as your brain restructures itself through the exercises you'll find in each chapter.

JUMP-START PLAN
STAGE 1: PRE-CONTEMPLATION

Chapter 6
This Is Your Brain On Diets

The Fattening Way to Lose Weight

I'm in a gorgeous beach house in Malibu, surrounded by television cameras, crew members, producers, and four delightful women who are the participants in a makeover reality show. The women have been living here for several weeks, being filmed as they go about the business of getting gorgeous. A dietitian prepares fresh meals custom-designed for each woman. A trainer comes to the house to supervise daily workouts. The program is just what most people would think of as an ideal weight-loss setup, and sure enough, it's making the overweight participants thinner, healthier, more physically fit.

And oh, yes, they're also on the verge of a bloody coup. So there's that.

I've come to this show late in the game, since it's my job to help the ladies transition to real life. Right off the bat, I notice that all of them show signs of clinical depression—which is sort of good, because if they weren't so demoralized, I think they would kill their producers. They skulk around the Malibu mansion, staring daggers at the TV personnel, murder in their hollow eyes. Plus, they've been cheating. Last night they were caught ordering pizza from a nearby fast-food restaurant. No one knows what other crimes they may have perpetrated.

"What's *wrong* with them?" a producer asks me. "You'd think they'd be grateful, or at least cooperative. Why would they break rules that are set up for their own good?"

"It's because of the way the brain and body react to food deprivation," I say. "See, when something severely limits our food intake, it triggers a psychological mechanism that . . . "

But the producer's not listening. Like most people, she's absolutely convinced that the recipe for weight loss is intention plus force. She truly believes that to help the makeover gals, she should police them more rigorously, watch them more closely, make it even more difficult for them to get food.

So I give up on the producers and go straight to the dieters themselves. While the cameramen are changing film, we hatch a whispered plot. The next day I send a "care package" by express mail. It's an assortment of board games and jigsaw puzzles, but all the boxes have false bottoms. In the hidden spaces I've packed as many cookies, chocolate, and other forbidden food items as I can. Am I trying to sabotage the women's weight loss? Absolutely not. I'm trying to salvage it. Bet on this: when you see parents basing a kid's allowance on the child's weight loss, or a TV guest announcing her weight-loss intentions to 10,000,000 viewers, you can be pretty darn certain the person in question will end up chubbier. A little evolutionary logic will show you why.

EXPLANATION: FAMINE BRAIN

FACT: Your brain is an astonishingly complex and powerful instrument specifically designed to keep you from losing weight. Your ancestors survived and reproduced because their bodies were incredibly good at conserving fuel as they scurried from cave to cave, seeking edible grubs and possible mates, all, unthinkably, without a single Starbucks within walking distance.

FACT: Because it is an evolutionary imperative, eating is highly rewarding at many levels. Our brains are so attuned to starvation that consuming food causes not only physical satiety, but psychological payoffs. Not eating food makes us hungry, but it also makes us afraid.

FACT: The only natural conditions under which a wild animal will go hungry while exercising strenuously are emergencies—predator attacks, famine, natural disaster, etc.

FACT: Such emergency conditions "turn on" all our psychological and physical responses to stress. This means that dietary restriction and strenuous exercise, especially in combination, cause the brain to fixate on finding food and comfort, while pumping out hormones that signal the body to lay in supplies by becoming more sedentary and storing fat. (Incidentally, this constant bath of stress hormones also leads to a host of awful degenerative diseases.)

FACT: As very socially dependent beings, we get massively stressed out not only by predators and disasters, but also by social conditions such as negative judgment, loss of status, disapproval, and so on. Such factors have been shown to cause sharp rises in stress hormones among various social primates (baboons, chimpanzees, Britney Spears, etc.).

FACT: Sustaining this kind of stress by setting up constraints and expectations that make you even more panicky about keeping your dietary rules triggers your body's famine responses. These responses are far stronger than conscious intention. They are your Survivor instincts: ultimately, they will outwit, outlast, and outplay your attempts to diet by willpower.

FACT: If you increase the pressure to lose weight by swearing before God to go hungry forever, promising on *Oprah* that you'll drop the pounds, or telling your spouse she/he can divorce you if you get above a certain weight, you escalate your stress responses until they make you want to eat everything in the nearest Krispie Kreme distribution outlet, including the cashier. They will also cause your personality to change, much as Linda Blair's character changed in *The Exorcist*.

In short, courting all this stress is *absolutely, positively guaranteed* to cause "Famine brain," the state of mind that is the polar (get it?) opposite of the state of mind you need to lose weight permanently and peacefully. You simply can't outwit Mother Nature.

STARVATION RATIONS

Consider a study published in 1950 by an epidemiologist at the University of Minnesota named Ancel Keys—a study that somehow never gets mentioned in diet books. Keys studied a group of young men who had never worried about their weight and who'd been screened to make sure they were very healthy. Perfect specimens, these guys were; fit, happy, mentally stable. For 6 months, they restricted their calorie intake by about 50 percent (this is less drastic than many weight-loss programs I've tried, and much less restrictive than the medically supervised fasts some dieters undergo).

After a few months, the men in this study had gone . . . what's the technical term . . . totally barking postal. They were obsessed with food, talking and thinking about it constantly, losing interest in everything else. They were chronically angry, depressed, apathetic, and anxious. They lost their sense of humor. Many began biting their fingernails, smoking, drinking so much coffee that the experimenters had to restrict them to 9 cups a day. They started hoarding, even stealing—not just food, but all sorts of objects. Their relationships suffered. Their hair fell out.

And then there was the bingeing. Several subjects began losing all control and snorking huge amounts of food, then spiraling down into guilt and self-loathing. Some vomited after binges. When the study ended, the bingeing got worse, not better. For months, many of the men ate between 8,000 and 10,000 calories a day. Many reported feeling *increased* hunger right after a binge. Check out this tidbit from the original study:

> Subject No. 20 stuffs himself until he is bursting at the seams, to the point of being nearly sick and still feels hungry; No. 120 reported that he had to discipline himself to keep from eating so much as to become ill; No. 1 ate until he was uncomfortably full; and subject No. 30 had so little control over the mechanics of "piling it in" that he simply had to stay away from food because he could not find a point of satiation even when he was "full to the gills." . . . "I ate practically all weekend," reported subject No. 26 . . . Subject No. 26 would just as soon have eaten six meals instead of three. (p. 847)

As if this weren't bad enough, the men's metabolic rate (the number of calories it took to sustain their body weight) had dropped an average of 40 percent, illustrating (as a later analyst put it) "the tremendous adaptive capacity of the human body and the intense biological pressure on the organism to maintain a relatively consistent body weight."

This is precisely what was happening to those four ladies in the Malibu reality show, which is why I sent them food. I felt drastic action was needed to stop the escalating starvation response that was already eroding their happiness, causing them to sneak, hoard, and binge. The men in the Keys study gradually returned to something like normal life (although many of them seemed to have permanent behavior problems) *because they stopped trying to restrict their own eating*. Chronic dieters like me, the Malibu Four, and, perhaps, you, may try to restrict our eating for decades on end.

Now that I've corrected the landscape of my brain by using 4-day win strategies, I don't have to restrict my eating, and I no longer suffer from famine-brain's physical and psychological symptoms. Most people assume I've always been thin. But oh, lord, do I remember the hell I imposed on myself by dieting through willpower. Even when I didn't succeed in losing weight, the pressure to eat less made my brain and body fight back like a wild thing. If you've dieted extensively, you, too, have probably wrought havoc on everything from your sex drive to your work performance. Force-based food restriction works for a while, but it always breaks down, and when it does, the starved dieter eats like there's no tomorrow. Try this:

EXERCISE: WATCH YOUR FAMINE BRAIN

As you know, our environment is chock-full of messages that in order to be considered truly beautiful, you must be a small bony object that might easily fit through a subway grate. For just a few minutes, I'd like you to focus your attention on the media messages that really get to you: magazine or TV images of zero-body-fat athletes, dancers, or models; medical reports about obesity and morbidity; the cruel jokes your brothers make about your thick ankles. Write a list of these things in the space below:

1. Messages that make me think I must lose weight: _____

_____

_____

Now, bring to mind the things you tell yourself when you're feeling especially corpulent—perhaps mild exhortations like, "You could stand to trim down," but more likely angry rants, like "You disgusting sack of blubber! No one will ever love you until you lose that hideous flab!" Write these things in the following space:

2. Things I tell myself to make sure I'll lose weight: _____

_____

_____

Now, read over the two lists above. Let these items fill your mind—the skinny models, the angry judgments, the self-hatred. Holding them in your thoughts, answer these questions:

3. With these thoughts in mind, what emotions do I feel?

_____

_____

4. Holding these thoughts in my mind, do I feel more or less desire
to eat?

_____

_____

You may have found that you lose all appetite, feeling carefree and
delighted during the times you're trying to lose weight through shame and
self-admonition. If so, just put this book down and stop eating until you
look like Nicole Richie (this will be especially impressive if you are male). If,
on the other hand, you are human, you probably just triggered your innate
reaction to threats of deprivation. Your brain and body react by giving the
order, "Code red, code red! Find fattening food and eat it all and store every
bit of it! NOW!"

If you're going to be an effortlessly thin person, this has got to change.
In the past, you've probably alternated restrictive regimens with out-of-control eating, more or less like the subjects in the Keys study. This is not
because you're a naturally fat person. Absolutely everyone is likely to develop
backlash, obsession, and overeating as a physiological response to deprivation. _Overeating and putting on fat is the normal psychological response to the
mere expectation of being chronically hungry._ Let me emphasize: not _being_
chronically hungry, merely _expecting_ to be.

Even if you haven't lost large amounts of weight, this pattern is very likely
ingrained into your brain. Just by reading this, you've already begun to change
that. The Malibu Four managed to avert disaster—as far as I know, they never
killed a producer—but just in case you've reached the level of biological panic
I saw when those poor women were at their most desperate, the following chapters will help heal the brain wounds you've innocently inflicted on yourself.

JUMP-START PLAN
STAGE 2: CONTEMPLATION

Chapter 10

The Most Important Weight-Loss Skill in the History of the Universe

From where I'm sitting, the most promising weight-loss strategies aren't new diets or more insistent exhortations to control ourselves, but the implications of new research on brain function, which shows that the command center in our heads can basically be changed by experience—a phenomenon called neuroplasticity. Where I'm sitting, by the way, is in an office chair at a clinic that offers "brain mapping." The folks who work here wire up people's heads, plug them into computers, and collect all sorts of real-time data about the electrical activity generated by their brains.

So far, my brain-mapping results indicate that I have serious attention deficit disorder, but compensate for it with astronomical anxiety. This explains why my day-to-day train of thought goes like this: *Look! A shiny object! What's that doing in the—oh my God, I forgot to [call the plumber/e-mail my editor/feed the children/dress myself]! I'd better get that done right awa—Hey, look! A shiny object!"*

Fortunately, neuroscience has recently determined that I can deliberately alter the way my brain works. So far, I've spent more than 10 hours in this chair, watching a line on the monitor that shows how vigorously my brain is producing beta waves, which are associated with anxiety. I'm "training down" my anxiety by doing whatever it takes to make that line drop. The process is hard to describe. I've found that the line goes down when I create a certain warm pressure in the middle of my head, but I can't tell you how I do it. Even so, I think it's working; I feel quite drunk with calm as my brain makes the adjustment. My anxiety has been much lower lately, in every situation. It feels fabulous. Though I have no earthly idea where I left my children.

My point is that we don't need to be doomed to corpulence just because our brains evolved to resist weight loss. We can out-think our own biology. However, as we've seen, simply imposing conscious will on our bodies won't work. It requires a new skill, one that's completely unfamiliar to most people and feels so subtle that we overlook its power: watching ourselves think, without getting caught up in our thoughts. And it's one we can acquire without leaving our own living room chairs.

EXPLANATION: RETROFITTING YOUR BRAIN

Jeffrey Schwartz, MD, is a psychiatrist who treats patients with obsessive-compulsive disorder (OCD). People who have OCD feel compelled to repeat behaviors like handwashing, even when they know it's excessive. If they don't wash their hands when the urge hits them, they feel incredibly high anxiety. Many psychologists use the classic diet advisor's "just stop it!" approach to treat these patients, forcing them to do things like hold dog feces without washing their hands. Surprise, surprise, this tends to be counterproductive. Most patients can defy their anxiety in the short term, but in the long run, they often backlash and become more compulsive than ever.

To Dr. Schwartz, this white-knuckle approach made no sense. He knew that on brain scans, people with OCD show unusually high activity in the part of the brain that triggers fear reactions. He could take pictures of this, MRI images that showed an electrically hyperactive spot in his patients' frontal lobes. He gave his patients these pictures of their brains overreacting. When the handwashing urge hit, Dr. Schwartz had them look at the MRIs and tell themselves, "It feels like I should wash my hand, but really, this is just an electrical impulse in my brain." Then they'd do something they enjoyed—Dr. Schwartz mentions gardening, though I prefer making crank telephone calls to elected officials—for 15 minutes.

At first, some of Dr. Schwartz's patients had to repeat this, but after a maximum of two 15-minute sessions, the urge to wash their hands had subsided. The longer they persisted with this exercise, the shorter the duration of their urges. Finally, the handwashing anxiety would stop. At that point, Dr. Schwartz took more MRI images—and found that the structure of his patients' "abnormal" brains had changed. Their brains were now structurally normal.

I believe (and early research suggests) that overeating is often a self-calming compulsion similar to OCD. When a handwasher gets psychologically stressed, say by the unsettling illness of a pet goldfish, that person's first reaction may be to crank up the faucets. For a compulsive eater like me, Mr. Fin's declining health would lead straight to a pound cake. Being barred from eating used to cause me enormous discomfort—not physical hunger, but the same freakout experienced by handwashers who can't get to the sink. For anyone who's ever been calorie-deprived by dieting, actual hunger can be terrifying. We can't overcome this by going on stricter diets, any more than an obsessive-compulsive handwasher can achieve normalcy by clutching dog poo.

The exercise you're about to learn will help you respond effectively to stress without having to eat anything. I believe that, in a process similar to the one Dr. Schwartz observed in his patients, *practicing the exercise repeatedly may alter the physical structure of your brain, so that you no longer feel any need to eat when you aren't hungry.* It's so subtle you may at first underestimate its power, but if it's the only thing you learn from this book, practicing it regularly can stop you from overeating.

This exercise will quietly remove you from Stage 1, the "pre-contemplative" state where most dieters are stuck, unconsciously, for most of their lives. Various versions of this practice exist in every culture that has a tradition of "contemplation." Contemplatives are people who stand back a step from the usual grimy struggle of human activity, seeing and thinking with unusual clarity. They're also the members of any given culture who can do extraordinary things, like staying calm in disasters, providing wisdom in times of crisis, accessing mystical states, and imagining Donald Trump with normal hair. You don't have to believe in shamanism to take advantage of the contemplatives' way of being. It can happen anytime you change your behavior by emerging from Stage 1, Pre-contemplation to Stage 2, Contemplation. This next lesson will teach you to become the kind of contemplative I call the Watcher.

EXERCISE: THE WATCHER, THE DICTATOR, AND THE WILD CHILD

In Chapter 6, I asked you to recall the set of controlling, bitter thoughts with which your mind tries to lash you to various weight-loss regimens. These words, like all verbal thinking, are produced by the computer-self. You saw how your creature-self reacts, by panicking and breaking the rules. In this chapter, we'll picture these rule-making and rule-breaking parts of you as humans. Tiny humans. We'll call them the Dictator and the Wild Child.

The instructions below may feel odd, but I want you to follow them anyway because of the way they affect your brain. First, hold out your right hand, palm up. Imagine a 2-inch-tall version of yourself in a military uniform, with a whip in one hand and a gun in the other, stomping around in your palm, shrieking deeply personal insults and commanding you to lose weight. This is the Dictator. Now hold up your left palm (you may have to put down this book for a minute) and picture your Wild Child there: 2 inches tall, dressed in skins and bark, covered with scars, waiting for an opportunity to escape or subvert the Dictator's brutal control. Watch until you can see them both clearly in your mind's eye.

Now, while watching these two mini-you's, I want you to see that as dysfunctional as they may be, both of them are essentially good. The Dictator wants you to be healthy and beautiful. It gets frantic about your weight for the same reason you might freak out if you saw a beloved pet wandering into traffic. It screams and yells, pens you in or drags you around—anything to keep you from a horrible fat fate. On the other hand, the Wild Child is the part of you that evolved to avoid starvation and captivity. It panics when the Dictator berates, shames, and tries to control it. It knows the Dictator is planning to starve it. So it's not surprising that the instant the Dictator is weakened by stress, hunger, or environmental chaos, the Wild Child leaps into action and eats like a junkyard dog.

Think through the well-meaning motivations of both your Dictator and your Wild Child, until you really understand that within their limited perspectives they're doing their very best. Then offer them both kindness. One useful method is to silently repeat these phrases from the classic "loving-kindness" meditation: *"May you be well. May you be happy. May you be free from suffering."* It may help to set the book aside again and close your eyes. Continue offering these good wishes while visualizing both the Wild Child and the Dictator until you genuinely mean it, until you can feel compassion toward both sides of yourself. When you get there, consider the following question.

Who are you?

The only reason you can "see" and offer kindness to both Dictator and the Wild Child is that you're not either one of them. You've moved into a third realm of consciousness, which resides, literally, in a different part of your brain. Call it the Watcher.

This is a subtle transition. You may feel it as a slight sense of loosening and relief, the psychological equivalent of taking off a tight, itchy piece of clothing. Or it might feel revolutionary, an epiphany that changes you permanently the first time you feel it. I've seen many people who do this exercise begin to cry—and these are individuals who've been through 17 kinds of hell without shedding a tear. Often, I get a specific sensation when someone near me moves into the Watcher-self. It's as though an enormous, powerful, invisible creature has slipped soundlessly into the room and settled itself against the wall. It raises every hair on my body.

You may not feel this at first, or it may be so inconspicuous that you don't even notice it. Just persist with the exercise, offering the Dictator and Wild Child best wishes for at least a full minute at a time (it often takes about 50 seconds for a beginner). When you can clearly imagine both sides of your dieting self, without identifying completely with either of them, consider another question:

Holding this mental position, how do you feel about food?

While both the Dictator and Wild Child make you want to overeat, your Watcher self is not nearly as compulsive. It doesn't feel either rigidly controlled or totally out-of-control. In fact, according to some medical psychologists, it's physiologically impossible for your mind to stay locked in a war of control when you're engaging its ability to generate compassion and appreciation. It is a place of great inner peace. Since it's also the only mindset from which you can make yourself an effortlessly lean person, I call it "the place of Thinner Peace." True, this is a roll-your-eyes pun, but it gives me a memorable label for a distinct inner sensation. I know from brain mapping that this is literally the feeling of my brain releasing anxiety.

THINNER PEACE: KEYS TO THE KINGDOM

I can't stress this strongly enough: Learning to access the place of Thinner Peace is *the most important weight-loss skill in the history of the universe,* and it will enable you to stay on any weight-loss regimen. And now that you've learned about and practiced the pre-contemplative and contemplative skills discussed in the preceding chapters, you're ready to integrate this crucial skill into your life.

Almost all of us assume there's only one way to lose weight: by willpower, by white-knuckle resistance, by forcing the body with an aggressive, adversarial, disciplinarian mind. This can be achieved *sometimes*, though not often. Maintaining it long-term? I don't think that can be done. I've seen numerous clients deploy incredible discipline, using their Dictator selves to trap, dominate, and starve their Wild Child selves. Losing weight this way is as draining as keeping a violent criminal pinned to the floor with sheer force. But even if you manage to do it, you can't hold your own Wild Child in a hammerlock for the rest of your life. The minute you get tired, distracted, or sick, the Dictator loses control, and the Wild Child goes into a feeding frenzy.

That's the whole reason I wrote this book. Simply going on a diet program, without changing your mental set, causes backlash and weight gain. *This is an inevitable reality, based on the way our brains and bodies are designed.* But if you use 4-day win techniques to become a Watcher and bring yourself to Thinner Peace, your brain changes, as well as your body. Weight loss happens without backlash or resistance.

The deceptively quiet power of this brain-shifting strategy has made it a favorite of contemplatives in many places, throughout time. Stepping back from the Dictator and the Wild Child and becoming the Watcher, is like thinking you've been stuck on a railroad track, able to move only backward and forward, and discovering that you had the capacity to fly all along. Even if this initially only feels like a tiny hop off the tracks, it can be the beginning of a whole new life. Becoming a Watcher is a forefield skill, one you'll want to use daily, or even several times a day, once you master it.

JUMP-START PLAN
STAGE 3: PREPARATION

Chapter 21
Eat Whatever The Hell You Want

Preparing to Eat Less

Derek, an orthopedic surgeon, got out of the shower one morning and noticed he was 80 pounds overweight. "I'd been ignoring it, rationalizing it, hiding it from myself," he told me later. "But that day I just looked at myself and thought, 'Holy crap, I'm fat!'" Derek had never dieted before, so he went out and got himself a weight-loss book: *The Zone Diet.* "It looked pretty reasonable to me," he said, "and it worked." That's all Derek ever needed. Now he's an Ironman triathlete, lean and chiseled as a greyhound. Once he came out of pre-contemplation, Derek needed very little information or structure to get fit and stay that way.

Sharon's weight vacillates by about 25 pounds. When it goes up, she vows to eat less and move more, but on her own, it never really tracks. So she goes to Jenny Craig, where food is provided and weekly counseling sessions with a personal, well-trained consultant eliminate the need to keep track of calories. This gives her enough structure to feel luxuriously cared for. She enrolls every 5 years or so and thinks of her Jenny Craig experiences as "a vacation from having to deal with my weight all by myself."

Anita is the vice president of a fairly large corporation. Her gift for leadership has made her plenty of money, and her quick mind has absorbed enormous amounts of knowledge. However, having two alcoholic parents left Anita with many emotional-eating tendencies, which used to make her weight zoom up and down like an extreme skier. She tried enrolling in over-eaters Anonymous, going on a medically supervised diet, and even hired her own health-food chef and personal trainer. These strategies always backfired when Anita came to see her support people as authority figures—just like her boozing parents. She'd become angry at these support people, just as she was angry at her parents, then violate the rules they'd set for her. Ultimately, she'd fire them.

As Anita worked with me, she realized that each time her Wild Child gulped a Twinkie or skipped an exercise session, she felt she'd finally triumphed over her parents. But she also felt like the fat kid who deserved her parents' neglect. The fix was for Anita to get out of EASY diet mind (getting an external authority as the expert) and into CALM mind (learning so much that she became the expert herself). She began reading up-to-the-minute diet research, then designed her own diet and exercise program. She still works with a chef and a trainer, but *she tells them what the program will be, not the other way around.* For someone with Anita's personality and psychological history, the combination of high structure and high information did the trick. She's lost 50 pounds and says she feels great.

I started dieting when I was 6. For the next 30 years or so, my choices about what, when, were, and how much to eat came from my brain, not my body—or anyway, that was the plan. I'd learn what the current expert had to say, memorize calorie lists, obtain all the chard or trout or bird seed or whatever else was allowed on that program. I'd restrict my eating to the times, places, amounts, and exact food combinations advised by the diet. All would go well until the polar bear effect would kick in and I'd binge my brains out on precisely the foods that were *dis*allowed by my diet du jour.

This process made me a walking calorie calculator. I can tell you the nutritional content of pretty much any food you throw at me (and you'll find that if you constantly tell people the nutritional value of what they're eating, they throw food at you quite a lot). However, I'm also allergic to intellectually based dietary restriction. Three decades of Dictator dominance turned my Wild Child into a rebel with a very clear cause: to eat whatever anyone, including my own mind, instructed me not to eat. Tell me, for example, that I can't have Ho-Ho's, and though I've never partaken of that particular delicacy, I will instantly become a Ho-Ho ho. Forbid carbs, and I'll put away a loaf of bread before you finish talking. Tell me to cut out fat, and I'll butter everything I swallow, including prescription medication.

So these days, I don't follow any diet program. I literally can't. I eat strictly according to appetite: whenever and whatever the hell I want. *But I do this from the position of my inner Watcher,* who isn't compulsive about food and isn't tempted by empty calories or excessive fullness. My one dietary discipline is to return, return, return to the place of Thinner Peace, and eat only in that state of mind. Ultimately, you'll be able to do this, too, with a high level of confidence that your real nature will choose to eat exactly what's right for you.

When I first gave up on dieting, my famine-damaged brain gravitated toward all the junk food I'd been telling myself not to eat. Gradually, as my brain healed, my Watcher self began asking me to eat healthy food, particularly fruit and veggies. But I always wanted nuts with the fruit and oily dressings or sauces on vegetables. Until yesterday, I thought I was being a little naughty with the high-fat condiments. But yesterday I read a new study that found oil is necessary to metabolize the beneficial elements of plant foods, increasing the absorption of antioxidants by a factor of 6 or 7. When I read this, I raised my fist in rebel's triumph. It turns out those food combinations appeal to me for good reasons, *reasons my body knew well before my brain.*

This is not to say that I'm a flawless eater or that if you just start frolicking naked through fields of extra-virgin wilted organic arugula blossoms, you'll never want to consume anything unwholesome for the rest of your life. Please. What I am saying is that if you become a contemplative, learning to eat according to your body's real appetites without the distortions of mental dietary restriction, you'll find that there's a wisdom in your cells far greater than all the vast sea of information scientists have amassed trying to figure out what diet is best for you.

KNOWING WHAT TO EAT: INFORMATION AND STRUCTURE

The Beck Diet (eating whatever the hell you want) works only if you have fully connected with your Watcher self and *made that self the sole author of your choices.* The truth, as people like Jesus and Rumi and Lao Tzu were always trying to explain, is within us. The Buddha, for example, tried living according to the rules of the rich, which made him fat, and then following the rules of the ascetics, which made him so thin you could throw him across the Indian Ocean by the leg. Finally he decided to toss out the rulebook and refer to nothing but his true nature, and for the rest of his life, he was apparently a middleweight on the Middle Way, healthy, vigorous, and vibrant into old age. As I'm sure Jesus would've been, if they hadn't nailed him to a tree for having the audacity to say that the truth is within us.

So I'd love it if you decided to spend several months just learning to access your Watcher-self, allowing your diet to gradually become healthier, as mine did. But I am also an impatient person, and I realize that you have that event to attend this weekend and then that other event in 3 weeks, and you *absolutely have to be thinner by then.* So you'll probably want to start eating less right now, according to some set of dietary rules you can learn and

follow. I view all such programs as crutches—the only diet skill you'll ultimately need is the ability to create inner calm—but there's nothing wrong
with using crutches if you're wounded. If you're a typical dieter, you're as
wounded as wounded can be. So let's find out what kind of diet program
will work best for you, starting right here and now.

EXPLANATION: HOW TO CHOOSE A FITNESS PROGRAM WHILE YOUR BRAIN HEALS

There are two components that determine whether a fitness program will
work for you: information and social structure. Different weight losers, at
different points in their lives, need different levels of each component. If you
have tons and tons of nutrition information between your ears, as I did by
the time I was an adult, you already have a pretty darn good idea what you
should eat to lose weight. You've probably been on diets that made you sick
and others that made you feel and look healthier, right up to the point where
you lost all vestiges of self-control. You know what combination and amount
of food works as a weight-loss program for you.

On the other hand, if you're new to dieting, you'll need to learn some
basic information, which you can get from innumerable books, magazines,
Web sites, and experts. I'll recommend a few in the following chapter, after
we've determined your diet profile. But remember this crucial point: *When
you turn to any external source for diet information, the goal is to internalize the
information so that you can make smart choices, not to see the external source as
the author of your decisions.* You can get fly-fishing instructions or information on postage stamps without putting your teacher on a pedestal, and the
same is true of weight loss. *Your ultimate goal is to become the expert who
decides what you eat.*

Besides information, you may also need an external social structure (one
or more people working with you) to support you in applying all that useful
diet information. We've talked a bit about limiting your time with the Munch
Bunch and the No-Go's and getting more involved with the Slender
Befrienders and Go-Go's. This helps your whole life become a fitness-friendly
social structure. But something more formal and targeted may be necessary
for you as you start losing weight. Some people are naturally comfortable
with high levels of structure. They easily and happily adapt to, say, attending

weight-loss support groups or having a nutritionist choose, prepare, and deliver their food every day. This gives them the feeling of being cared for, maybe even pampered (it would give me a feeling of violent rage). There's no right or wrong way to feel about structure, but it's important that at any given point on your journey toward permanent skinniness, you stay embedded in the kind of structure that works best for you.

I'm going to restate the key fact I just told you to remember about information, because it can't be overemphasized: If you choose a highly structured weight-loss program, *remember that participating in this structure is your free choice. Never see yourself as the servant of the structure. See yourself as allowing it to serve you.*

For example, I had one client, Maureen, who got her weight under control by attending Overeaters Anonymous. She was a rabid True Believer, who constantly referred to OA's rules and regulations. She saw herself as "obeying" the structure and having no personal volition. There was an almost cultlike quality to her devotion. After a few months of this, her Wild Child took over, trying to help her grow up and achieve psychological independence. She began bingeing, then punishing herself for being bad. She was caught in a childlike role, seeing her program as a parent figure: "Do your chores, little girl, and you'll get your reward." On the other hand, I've had several clients who decided to let OA *work for them* ("I'm a grown-up, but I need company and information") with impressive success.

If you do feel a need for some structure to play "good parent" and teach you to eat better, that's fine, *as long as you observe this need from the position of the inner Watcher.* We all begin as children, and even adults learn better by assuming a child ego state. But we also yearn for independence and authenticity. Our souls and bodies hate the well-meaning lie that says we have no choice but blind obedience. Ultimately, we separate from even the most benevolent and well-advised structure, internalizing the set of rules that works best for us. This is called growing up, and it's necessary for permanent weight loss. But there's no rush.

As you internalize information and gain confidence from structured systems, you'll be like a child learning to walk. You'll fall occasionally. Then you can check with the system to figure out why. You'll implement the methods they advise and *accept or reject all strategies depending on whether they resonate with your sense of what is working for your body, mind, and heart.* All information and structure, including the words you're reading now, are meant to help you find your balance until you learn to walk on your own. You will. And at that point, you won't need either information or structure as crutches. You'll still be able to learn from them, but you won't depend on them.

EXERCISE: YOUR CURRENT DIET PROFILE

Depending on your personality and past experience, you'll fall into one of four categories in choosing a diet and exercise program. The quiz below will help determine where you fall in the structure/information matrix. There are no right or wrong answers, and your responses may well change as the years go by. Just be honest now, so that you can steer toward the best way to lose weight by the time that event comes along, in just 3 weeks.

QUIZ: What's Your Diet Profile?

Answer the following true-false questions as honestly as possible. There is no wrong answer to any of the questions.

1. TRUE   FALSE   I'm not confident enough to be a real do-it-yourselfer; I'm very happy leaving difficult jobs to the experts.

2. TRUE   FALSE   It's hard for me to face a difficult task without support from someone knowledgeable and kind, who can give me feedback and encouragement.

3. TRUE   FALSE   When it comes to learning a new skill, I'd prefer to work with a flesh-and-blood instructor or teacher as opposed to a book or instructional video.

4. TRUE   FALSE   No matter what I'm undertaking, I feel safer and more motivated when I have someone to coach me through unfamiliar tasks.

5. TRUE   FALSE   I don't want to have to keep track of things like calories, fat grams, minutes of exercise, and so on. I have too many things on my mind as it is.

6. TRUE   FALSE   I like working with people, but I also like to know why they do what they do. When I go to

the doctor, get my car fixed, or hire a repair-
man to work on my home, I want to know
exactly what they're doing and why.

7. TRUE   FALSE   I don't like to work alone, and I don't like being
a subordinate. I generally work in teams where
I'm the one who really understands what needs
to be done and how the team should function.

8. TRUE   FALSE   I'm a natural-born leader. I like taking charge,
because I usually understand what's going on
better than the people around me.

9. TRUE   FALSE   If money were no object, I'd much rather pay
someone to give me a pedicure, do my hair, or
decorate my living space than do the work
myself—but I want to make all the decisions
about how the job gets done.

10. TRUE   FALSE   I don't have time or patience to perform everyday, routine tasks; I prefer to hire help or del-
egate the labor for these tasks so I can focus on
more interesting challenges.

11. TRUE   FALSE   I love figuring out complicated things on my
own. I want to know how everything works,
and I get impatient unless I get to direct my
own learning process.

12. TRUE   FALSE   It's frustrating for me to work in teams; when
I'm trying to achieve a goal, I'd rather go at my
own pace than have to coordinate with other
people.

13. TRUE   FALSE   I love to get information (from books, experts,
TV shows, any source) that explains how the
world works in detail.

14. TRUE   FALSE   When I'm passionate about a subject, nothing
can stop me from learning everything there is
to know about it. I'm almost obsessive.

15. TRUE   FALSE   If you gave me a choice between having an
expert do something for me and learning to do
it myself, I'd almost always choose the do-it-
myself option.

16. TRUE   FALSE   I'm highly self-motivated, and I don't need to know every detail about whatever I'm attempting. Just tell me some basic rules, leave me alone, and let me work!

17. TRUE   FALSE   I like simple, clear goals, and left to my own devices, I'll attain them. Having to involve other people in any effort frustrates me.

18. TRUE   FALSE   I like functioning in systems where there's an established way to do things (for example: the school system, a company, a family tradition, the military). I've earned individual recognition for excelling in such environments.

19. TRUE   FALSE   Give me a job, and I'll get it done if you stay out of my way. Period.

20. TRUE   FALSE   If I believe in what I'm doing, I go straight into action without waiting for anyone else to come along, and I don't stop until I've achieved my objectives.

SCORING

If most of your True responses showed up in questions 1 through 5, you fit what I call the Apprentice profile. You need high structural support, but not all that much detailed information. Sharon, the Jenny Craig dieter, is an Apprentice.

If your True answers clustered in questions 6 through 10, you fit the profile of a VIP. You learn a lot about what you want to accomplish, then coordinate people to implement strategies you design. Anita, the CEO with the alky parents, is a VIP dieter.

Getting a lot of True responses on questions 11 through 15 means you have a Scholar profile. High information, not much structure. After my years of diet insanity, I ended up a diet Scholar.

Finally, if you got a lot of True answers on questions 16 through 20, you're an Explorer. You need a few good instructions, a lot of space, and a clear goal but little information, and little structure.

The chart on the next page will tell you how to go about starting your weight-loss diet, depending on your needs for information and structure at this point in your life.

HIGH NEED FOR INFORMATION

HIGH NEED FOR STRUCTURE

THE VIP ARCHETYPE (EXAMPLE: ANITA)

How to Proceed:

Get any or all of the books you'll see listed in the "High Need for Information" section. Then, connect to any or all of the systems listed in the "High Need for Structure" section. Sign up for one or more of these systems (you could have both a dietitian and a trainer, for instance), depending on your resources and preferences. *Always remain the designer and administrator of your diet plan. Stay in your Watcher self to continually connect to your power and keep you from backlashing.*

HIGH NEED FOR INFORMATION

LOW NEED FOR STRUCTURE

THE SCHOLAR ARCHETYPE
(EXAMPLE: MARTHA)

How to Proceed:

Get any or all of the books you'll see listed in the "High Need for Information" section. Read them, compare the information from different sources, and see what sounds sensible and appealing to you. If you want any structure at all, connect to a "Low Need for Structure" system. Better yet, design your own weight-loss diet. *Stay in your Watcher space as you learn, testing every new piece of information against your own logic and knowledge, instead of enslaving yourself to an intellectual idea of righteous eating.*

LOW NEED FOR INFORMATION

HIGH NEED FOR STRUCTURE

THE APPRENTICE ARCHETYPE
(EXAMPLE: SHARON)

How to Proceed:

Get ideas from friends, magazines, newspaper articles, or TV about a weight-loss program you might like—maybe one of the systems I've listed in the "High Need for Structure" section. Once you've chosen a system, get connected to it right away. Read whatever material is required by your program, but let the system do the work. *Do not make the mistake of thinking this condition should last forever. Your Watcher self will tell you that apprenticeship is the path to mastery, and your goal is to internalize and own the rules you are learning from the system.*

LOW NEED FOR INFORMATION

LOW NEED FOR STRUCTURE

THE EXPLORER ARCHETYPE
(EXAMPLE: DEREK)

How to Proceed:

Go online, ask trusted friends, or see your doctor to find out which diet books and systems they think would work for you. Any of the books I've listed under "Low Need for Information" could work. Alternatively, you could enlist in one of the "Low Need for Structure" systems, making sure the one you choose feels right. Familiarize yourself with the rules, and get going! *Stay connected to the place of Thinner Peace so that you know if something's off kilter—if the system or information you're relying on may need to be checked, revised, or traded for something better.*

SOME RECOMMENDED DIETS
FOR EACH PROFILE

Given the guidelines in the chart on page 330, there are still infinite diet options available to every weight-loss wannabe. I have a few favorites, based on what I've seen recommended by physicians, nutritionists, and medical researchers I respect, and what has worked for my clients and myself at different times in my life. Below you'll find some recommendations for books, Web sites, and systems. You can utilize any of them or any other resource as long as they provide a level of information and social support you like.

People who want high information tend to drawing their diet strategies from written material, the more detailed, the better. They'd rather not have a lot of face-time with an advisor. People who like lots of structure prefer flesh-and-blood information sources to printed ones. I've included both human and written components in the recommendations below.

BOOKS FOR PEOPLE
WITH HIGH NEED FOR INFORMATION
(VIP'S AND SCHOLARS)

All these books have corresponding Web sites, with updated information. Check 'em out when you crave new data. Also, log on to sites like the American Medical Association's nutrition information or the latest news stories on diets (popular media cover really interesting studies, weeding out the less interesting and giving you the hints you need to Google the latest findings).

> *Ultrametabolism*, by Mark Hyman
> *8 Weeks to Optimum Health* and *Eating Well for Optimum Health*, by
>   Andrew Weil, MD
> *The Way to Eat*, by David Katz, MD
> *Eat More, Weigh Less*, by Dean Ornish, MD
> *The South Beach Diet*, by Arthur Agatston, MD
> *The Sonoma Diet*, by Connie Guttersen
> *French Women Don't Get Fat*, by Mireille Guiliano
> *The Zone Diet*, by Barry Sears
> Pritikin Program books, by Robert Pritikin
> Mediterranean diet (go online to find research from many different
>   authors)

Glycemic Index diet (multiple sources; see Christiane Northrup's online newsletter)

BOOKS FOR PEOPLE WITH LOW NEED FOR INFORMATION (APPRENTICES AND EXPLORERS)

Get one that looks doable, and do it. If you're an Explorer, you'll base your diet on the book you choose. If you're an Apprentice, you don't have to read anything; just sign on to a good system and let your advisors teach you to eat well.

Dieting for Dummies, by Jane Kirby, RD
8 Minutes in the Morning, by Jorge Cruise
The South Beach Diet for Beginners, online
Get With the Program, by Bob Greene
Body For Life, by Bill Phillips
Fat Loss 4 Idiots online information resources

SYSTEMS FOR PEOPLE WITH HIGH NEED FOR STRUCTURE (VIP'S AND APPRENTICES)

These are just a few systems that are easy to locate nationwide. Your doctor, local health clinic, or independent weight-loss centers may be good, too. Don't be the system's slave; choose one to *work for you, not vice versa.*

Jenny Craig (the highest-touch, most thoroughly supportive program out there for people who aren't zillionaires but are willing to invest in their health and need systems to do it)

Weight Watchers (not quite as high-touch as Jenny Craig; food available, but not required; less expensive but also more work)

Overeaters Anonymous (very rigid structure, lots of personal contact, and it's free!)

Personal chef services (many programs are surprisingly affordable; check the internet and your Yellow Pages)

eDiets (an excellent service that helps you personalize your plan online; will help you structure an eating program around just about any diet out there; lacks the face-to-face contact with real people that you may need, especially at first)

SYSTEMS FOR PEOPLE
WITH LOW NEED FOR STRUCTURE
(SCHOLARS AND HEROES)

Try any of these. Or not. Ideally, you'll either design your own program (if you're a Scholar) or pick a decent one and just do it (if you're an adventurer.) Or, you could choose not to use any system at all, just act on what you know.

> The Beck Diet (eat whatever the hell you want, but only from a mental place of Thinner Peace)
> Any buddy system (have friends lose weight along with you, or bet a pal you can drop weight)
> The Oprah "Spa Girls" plan (read about setting up a weight-loss group on Oprah's Web site)
> Online program of your choice (browse at will, pick anything interesting, try it on for size)
> SlimFast (buy the shakes, follow the plan)

READ CHAPTER 32 OF THIS BOOK TO HELP
YOU IMPLEMENT THE DIET YOU CHOOSE

To start losing weight immediately, choose a diet method that fits your profile, and find out (either by getting information or signing up for a program) what the recommended menu is. Then, set up a 4-day win, eating according to your new diet rules for 4 days. Of course, you might link many 4-day wins to lose all the weight you want, *but the first 4 days are by far the hardest, and if you can hang on that long, you'll feel less deprived, see early signs of weight loss, and get some momentum that will take you a long way toward persistence and success.*

You may be a little hungry during your first 4-day win, depending on what diet you choose and how you're used to eating. No matter what your program suggests, do not let yourself get ravenous. Before you start dieting, please read Chapter 6, on how to eat a bit less without going into famine brain! Otherwise, you'll end up fatter than ever. By using the techniques in Chapter 32 as you begin following your chosen diet, you can actually stay on the plan and lose weight—permanently.

"Eat Whatever the Hell I Want" 4-Day Win

Ridiculously Easy Daily Goal: *For the next 4 days, I'll spend 10 minutes a day checking out the weight-loss programs listed in this chapter. I'll either look them up online, talk to friends, call local agencies, or go to the bookstore and browse through the Diet section. Then I'll pick a program. I'll go on to read Chapters TK and TK of this book, so that I can design my first "eat less" 4-day win.*

Small Daily Reward: _____

_____

Slightly Larger 4-Day Reward: _____

_____

	Dates of My Current 4-Day Win	Check Off Completed Days Here
Day 1:	___/___/___	_____
Day 2:	___/___/___	_____
Day 3:	___/___/___	_____
Day 4:	___/___/___	_____

If you're already on a weight-loss regimen, remember that the 4-day win will enhance it, not conflict with it. If you know what to do, this program will help you do what you know. Feel free to stay on any weight-loss program while you learn 4-day win skills!

JUMP-START PLAN
STAGE 4: ACTION

Chapter 32
I Will Fight No More (And Eat A Bit Less) Forever

Actually Losing Weight

The Pima Indians of Gila Valley, close to my own Arizona home, have a hell of a time losing weight. Of course, this wasn't true for most of the 2,000 years the Pima inhabited Gila Valley. As desert farmers, they ate native plants like squash and beans, and low-fat meat from rabbits and birds. They also underwent many periods of famine, and so (according to some researchers) the Pima experienced a lot of selective pressure that favored a so-called "thrifty gene" (the human leptin receptor gene is a prime suspect). This gene helped their bodies store fat very quickly in times of plenty, so as to live through times of want.

Then, in the 1920s, the natural water supply flowing through the Gila Valley was diverted for use by farmers who were not of Pima origin (three guesses which racial group these interlopers represented). To keep the Pima from starving in their now-permanently drought-stricken homeland, the U.S. government began giving the tribe food, such as lard, cheese, and white flour. The results were disastrous. Today, at least half of the adults in the Gila Valley Pima community are obese, and 80 percent of those people have Type II diabetes.

Dr. Eric Ravussin has been studying the Pima since 1984. At one point, he trekked to a remote part of the Sierra Madre mountains in Mexico to visit a group of Pima who have the same genetic profile as the Arizona group, but live and eat in more traditional ways. The Mexican Pima studied by Dr. Ravussin weren't overweight, and only three had diabetes. His conclusion? "[I]f the Pima Indians of Arizona could return to some of their traditions, including a high degree of physical activity and a diet with less fat and more starch, we might be able to reduce the rate, and surely the severity, of unhealthy weight in most of the population,"

In other words, even if your genetic deck is stacked against you, it's still very possible to be lean and healthy if you (here it comes) eat less, move more. Surprise, surprise.

EXPLANATION: THE BOTTOM LINE FOR KEEPING YOUR BOTTOM IN LINE

I mention the Pima because their experience points out that people really do have distinctly, even dramatically different hereditary tendencies when it comes to getting fat. There are about 340 genes involved in determining your weight, and only identical siblings share exactly the same genetic profile, including its specific tendencies to be chubbier or leaner. Even if you don't have Pima ancestry, there are probably lots of people in the world who really can eat more than you do, while exercising less, and still be skinny.

This is not fair.

It is absolutely not fair. It is terribly, hideously, inexcusably unfair. It is so unfair that the government, the pope, the army, and God omnipotent really should do something to change it . . . which is probably what a bunch of people who starved to death in the Middle Ages thought about your ancestors being able to survive on so very little gruel. Hey, you win some, you lose some. So, unjust though it may be, we're going to work with your metabolism. That means eating fewer calories than you burn in order to lose weight, and you can do it.

If you're not eating much, but the weight isn't budging, you need to: 1) repair your brain so that it allows your metabolism to correct itself; and possibly 2) eat even less.

THIS IS SO &*#@ UNFAIR!

But, like so many American Indian tribes, a legacy of injustice is part of our history. Fighting what is, especially in our own genetic makeup, is a no-win proposition. Like Chief Joseph of the Nez Perce, all of us might want to reach the point where we say, "I will fight no more forever." Instead of being angry at our chubby genes, we can learn to be healthy by accepting our biological reality and adapting our way of life, like the Mexican Pima, so that we never have to be overweight.

FINDING JUSTICE IN 4 DAYS

The best way to tolerate the injustice is to remember what I heard, over and over, from people who had successfully lost a lot of weight and kept it off:

> "I was only hungry for the first 4 days."
> "I didn't notice it after 4 days."
> "It was fine after the 4 days or so."
> "The first 4 days were tough; after that, not bad."

This book is called *The 4-Day Win* because I want you to remember that you don't have to sustain a state of ravenous starvation for the rest of your life to be lean. In fact, that will inevitably make you fat. Just because you have a tendency to gain weight doesn't mean nature "wants you" to be extra large, any more than the Arizona Pima are "meant to" suffer from obesity and diabetes. If you're currently used to eating 10,000 calories a day, if you're using food as a calming drug, or have a naturally inefficient metabolism, losing weight will mean eating a lot less, and tolerating some hunger, sometimes. *But the sense of deprivation must be mild, never severe, and it should never last longer than 4 days.*

You're going to use 4-day wins, along with every single skill I've mentioned in this book, as you reduce your calorie intake enough to ensure you burn off extra weight, forever. Let's review a few of the main points, then get specific about how you, personally, are going to eat so much less that your excess body fat will become a distant memory.

- Learn to think of your body as a wary prey animal, a creature that doesn't respond well to force, anger, control, attack, sudden moves, or starvation. Learn to love your creature-self.
- Notice the difference between gut hunger and brain hunger. The first condition requires food. The second requires fixing a disordered craving pattern.
- Do not go to war on yourself or your appetite. Instead, access the part of your brain where only compassion and observation can occur—not fear, conflict, or compulsiveness. Become the Watcher any time you feel out of control, to structurally repair your brain.

- Habitually question all of your own thoughts that cause anxiety. Look for reasons they may not be true—because they aren't. Seeing that they are not true quiets the terrible stress created by your own mind, without making you eat.

- Become your own research project. Correlate events in your past with times when you became fatter or thinner, and notice which activities, people, and places in your present life cause you to feel like a rat in a trap.

- Get used to continually building a life that meets your real needs, desires, and destiny. By eliminating "rat trap" components and adding "rat park" elements, you'll create a life free from craving, including the craving for excess food.

- Experiment with different food combinations to see which foods satisfy you most while padding your rump the least. Focus on natural, unprocessed foods with simple flavors. Eat what you know your body wants.

- Make sure you aren't in a state of exhaustion (possible adrenal burnout). If you are, begin resting and relaxing more until you actually want to exert effort of some kind.

- Note your daily patterns of action (your daymap), and begin using your circadian rhythm to change the pattern each day, so that you end up in the right place to exercise more than you've done in the past. Repeat each new behavior on 4 consecutive days to establish your new daymap.

- Modify your daymap so that your body expects food only at the healthiest times.

There's just one skill set you have yet to learn—and you're about to learn it. In this chapter, we'll talk about: 1) reducing your eating to weight-loss levels without creating famine brain; 2) keeping your food at a level that ensures continued weight loss; and 3) *never getting fat again*. With all the skills you have, plus those you're about to learn, YOU CAN DO IT!

THE MOTHER OF ALL EXERCISES: BACKING OFF THE CHUCK WAGON

STEP 1: NOTICE HOW MUCH FOOD YOU TYPICALLY EAT DURING AN AVERAGE DAY

Start with your eating daymap, and possibly your food-mood-brood journal. Notice how much you typically eat. You'll need some way to make some rough calculation of your food intake. If you're on a diet you've found in a book or article, these sources will list the type and amount of food you're supposed to eat at each meal. If you're a calorie-counting type, go ahead and use calories as your measure. If you're on a program like Jenny Craig, the portions are already designed for you, and your counselor can help you adjust your food intake as you observe how your body reacts to the program. I've never met any weight-struggling person who didn't have some system of food-intake measurement. Use what works best for you.

STEP 2: REDUCE YOUR DAILY FOOD INTAKE BY ABOUT 100 CALORIES PER DAY

Again, your formal diet book or diet advisor can tell you how much food equals about 100 calories. You may decide to cut out the least healthy food on your menu, throw away a certain percentage of food at each meal, cut back on simple carbs like refined-flour bread, pie crust, and jawbreakers, or replace a very rich food with something that's less rich but still satisfying. *Don't cut out any of your favorite foods unless they are immediately lethal. Work on developing abundance brain by reminding yourself that you can always have these foods, just not to the point of feeling horribly stuffed, getting fat, and making yourself sick.*

Sustain this new level of food intake (about 100 calories a day less than you're used to) for 4 days. The entire time, stay in the middle of your "hunger range." If 0 equals stuffed to the gills, and 10 equals ravenous, you want to stay right in the middle. Ideally, don't let yourself get hungrier than a 6 or more full than a 4 (3 and 7 are acceptable, but risky). *Never let your hunger get above an 8; this creates famine brain.* It's better to slightly raise your intake to stay below an 8 on the hunger scale for this 4-day win. If you do this, you'll be able to handle eating less without hunger during your next 4-day win.

STEP 3: SUBSTITUTE INEDIBLE NOURISHERS (SIN) EVERY TIME YOU REDUCE YOUR FOOD INTAKE, AND AFTER EVERY MEAL OR SNACK

Don't make the mistake of trying to live some gulag lifestyle without either food or comfort. As you reduce calorie intake, increase the amount of time you spend feeding your soul. At the conclusion of every meal or snack, give yourself 5 to 15 minutes of nonfood pleasure, in any legal fashion you choose. Use relaxation and breathing exercises, "treasuring" visualizations, sights, smells, sounds, and memories that remind you of love and happiness. Focus on your passions or hobbies, from spoon-hanging to shopping to learning about tectonic plate theory.

For 4-day win treats, indulge your inner Wild Child like a doting grandmother. SIN, SIN, SIN, to let your whole self know you're loved, catalyze the production of feel-good hormones, and give yourself infinite nonfood options for calming and delighting yourself at every level. This will help you tolerate the slight hunger you'll feel for 3 days. On the 4th day, you'll feel less physically hungry.

PROPER ZONE FOR HUNGER DURING WEIGHT LOSS

Never let yourself get uncomfortably full or miserably hungry. As you reduce calories, 4 days at a time, you will feel more and more satisfied on less food with each 4-day win.

When your body is hungry, eat until satisfied. If your brain is hungry, or you can't eat enough to feel satisfied, use brain-calming strategies instead of food. This will take practice and experience, and *you won't to do it perfectly. That's okay. Just do it.*

| 0 | 1 | 2 | 3 | 4 | 5 | 6 | 7 | 8 | 9 | 10 |

| Stuffed | Ideal Hunger Zone | Ravenous |

STEP 4: IF YOU'RE NOT LOSING WEIGHT, DROP YOUR FOOD INTAKE BY ABOUT ANOTHER 100 CALORIES PER DAY (AS CALCULATED BY YOU, YOUR DIETITIAN, A DIET BOOK, OR A WEIGHT-LOSS COUNSELOR)

As you keep lessening your food intake, you might feel a little hungry even if you're not losing weight yet. That's simply because your circadian rhythm is used to eating more than you actually need—and storing the extra food on your abundant pot belly. By reducing food gradually, adding nonfood nourishment, and giving your circadian rhythm 4 days to establish new expectations, you'll allow your body to stop wanting excessive food.

STEP 5: WATCH AND DEAL MENTALLY WITH ANY DEMONS THAT EMERGE INTO CONSCIOUSNESS, NOW THAT YOU'RE NOT USING FOOD AS A DRUG TO KEEP THEM REPRESSED

The mild hunger you may feel during the first 3 days of reduced food intake may scare you (actual hunger, however slight, is deeply unnerving to someone who has suffered repeated starvation). The fact that you aren't medicating your emotions with food may *terrify* you. All the demons you've been burying under baby-back ribs will emerge as you begin eating less and losing weight.

Bring out your food-mood-brood journal, and observe all sensations as well as thoughts. Watch any anxious mind-stories associated with the fear of future hunger, or of failing, or of succeeding, or that you'll be attacked by your deranged uncle, that no one has ever really loved you, that you have no talent, that your spouse is cheating, that your kids are going to disappear and never even visit you at the big-city bus station where you may spend your so-called "golden" years, even though you don't see anything golden about aging, which reminds you that you should bleach your teeth, because your high-school reunion is coming up and you're going to be the fat, yellow-toothed butt (BIG butt) of every joke, just like you were that time when in middle school when your physical education teacher yada yada yada yada *yada*.

In other words, the slight hunger you'll feel on the first 3 days of your 4-day win is a wonderful opportunity to examine your mind and address its dysfunctions, so that as you lose weight you'll become a happier and calmer person, not just a temporarily skinny food addict. Notice the stories that rise into your mind in the absence of food, go into the Watcher mode, and gently question each thought that causes anxiety. Are you certain your story is real, or is it just a tale told by an idiot, full of sound and fury, signifying nothing? No offense, but I think you'll find that the latter description fits reality better.

A final note on anxiety: *Remember that feeling frantic to lose 50 pounds by tomorrow is an anxious thought, and will keep you overweight.* Don't fight such thoughts, just observe them and offer yourself compassion. I'm not telling you this in order to force patience or to trap you in hell. I'm asking you to allay your own anxiety about rapid weight loss as well as everything else, because *this approach changes your brain into the brain of a skinny person.*

STEP 6: USE FLAVOR TRICKS TO LOWER YOUR HUNGER LEVEL (AND POSSIBLY YOUR FAT SET-POINT)

You'll feel a lot less hungry, and think about food less, if you use flavor tricks. Eat food with less intense or complex flavors—for example, real chicken instead of chicken that's been injected with sugar water, or oatmeal instead of a prepared oat cereal that's been engineered to increase your appetite by combining all sorts of flavors that you won't even notice—but which teach your brain to beg for more than you need.

As I said in Chapter 24, I've found that I can cut my appetite dramatically by using "flavor fasts," going an hour with no flavor of any kind, consuming a small amount of food that's high in calories but has no flavor (such a tasteless fish oil capsules) and then going another hour without flavors. This won't change any psychological hunger you might feel, but it may teach your brain to lower your hunger levels, and even your fat set point. Plus, most nutritionists highly recommend fish oil as a daily supplement; check with your doctor to make sure it's right for you.

STEP 7: KEEP CUTTING BACK ON FOOD, GRADUALLY, 4 DAYS AT A TIME, UNTIL YOU NOTICE A CHANGE IN YOUR BODY

If you continue edging your food intake down, you'll find that after a certain 4-day win (the one that takes you below the amount of food necessary to sustain your current weight) your body seems different. Even if you don't see much difference on your bathroom scale (yet), your clothes will be a little looser. You'll feel a little stronger, more mobile, more agile. The fat deposits on your body will begin losing fullness, like a balloon with the air leaking slowly away. This feeling, even more than the number on the scale (which may change due to water retention) is what tells you that you're losing weight.

STEP 8: LINK FIVE 4-DAY WINS TOGETHER
TO MAKE WEIGHT LOSS COMPLETELY HABITUAL

Once you're 4 days into a weight-loss routine, the hard part is over. Maintain your eating at this level, and even though you'll keep losing weight, you won't feel like you're on some brutal, skin-of-your-teeth regimen. Losing weight will be normal, like walking your dog, talking to your children, driving to work, or washing the dishes—not completely free of effort, but so familiar and habitual that it certainly doesn't feel difficult. Once you've linked enough 4-day wins to add up to 21 days of dieting (five wins plus 1 day) research indicates that your new way of life will be a habit that's actually hard to break.

FINALLY: BE NICE TO YOURSELF

Once you're in the swing of your weight loss, feeling and seeing the fat disappear, knowing that you can keep losing weight without suffering, and exchanging your mental demons for Thinner Peace, you'll experience a steady rise in your optimism and sense of efficacy. This is the "early win" that development theorists have found results in permanent positive change. You are not becoming a skinny caterpillar—a thinner version of the old you. You're becoming a whole new animal, a gorgeous airy thing that will never return to caterpillar life.

To sustain this wonderful process, just remember not to fly too high, too fast. Get lots of rest. Never forget to give yourself the daily rewards, or the bigger rewards you "win" every 4 days. Keep your food intake level at a weight-loss level, but never let your body get ravenous. Never give in to the temptation to starve or overwork your body. If you're impatient, and find yourself wanting to starve or overwork yourself, return to the identity of the Watcher, observe your Dictator insisting on harmfully harsh tactics, and gently remind all parts of yourself that at any given moment, everything is okay.

Paradoxically, this loving acceptance of yourself, at every moment of your weight loss experience, is what fuels the process of metamorphosis. It's the way you clear a path to a slim, lean body no matter what genetic pattern you inherited from your ancestors, so that you'll naturally fight your own body no more, and eat a bit less, forever.

JUMP-START PLAN
STAGES 5, 6, AND 7:
MAINTENANCE, RELAPSE,
AND TERMINATION

I'd love to give you the quick-and-dirty "jump-start" way to stay on your fitness program, get thin, and stay that way forever. Sadly, there isn't one. Nor is there an effective way to deal with weight-gain relapses, or to "terminate" your chubbiness, without re-structuring your whole way of being into that of a naturally thin person. How fortunate that you are holding in your very hands a primer that can teach you how to do these things! Coincidence? I think not.

Now that you've jump-started a weight loss program, just stay on your diet, linking 4-day wins. Your weight loss may fluctuate, depending on hormonal changes, water retention, and so on, but if you keep eating a bit less than necessary to sustain your larger weight, you'll usually notice perceptible weight loss (looser clothes, more muscle definition, easier time getting in and out of the car, people commenting) every 4 days.

So, while you're doing that, go back to Chapter 4 and finish reading this entire book. You'll find 4-day win explanations and exercises for dealing with any problems you may encounter as you lose weight. Learning these "backfield skills" will make your weight loss more and more natural, overcome the old barriers to sustained slenderness that have stopped you in the past.

If you find a strategy that seems appealing, internalize it through 4 consecutive days of practice. This will mean learning a new skill while sustaining your basic 4-day win of eating a bit less, staying on your fitness program. Don't panic! These skills will complement and enhance your weight loss, and none of them imposes any heavy burdens on your time or energy.

Your weight loss program will work best if you learn and practice all the skills, using "forefield" practices all the time, and "backfield" skills when you run into a particular problem and need to fix it. Learning them all is what turns simply weight loss into metamorphosis, makes you a butterfly instead of a thinner caterpillar, gives you a steadily increasing, gentle confidence in your body, your mind, and the communication between them. You can return to any of these Jump-Start skills whenever you want. But as you become more and more used to each practice and skill in this book, you'll find yourself simply thinking and acting as a thin person. Forever. Four little days at a time.

ABOUT THE AUTHOR

Martha Beck, PhD, is a Harvard-educated life coach and monthly columnist for *O, The Oprah Magazine*. She is the author of the bestsellers *Finding Your Own North Star: Claiming the Life You Were Meant to Live* and the memoir *Expecting Adam*. She lives in Phoenix, Arizona, with her family. Her hobbies include excessive viewing of the Discovery Channel, occasional pondering, and naps.

She can be contacted at www.MarthaBeck.com.